Emergent Care of the Burn Victim

Irving Feller, M.D.
Clinical Professor of Surgery,
University of Michigan Medical Center
Director of Michigan Burn Center

Claudella Archambeault-Jones, R.N.
Director of Education
National Institute for Burn Medicine

Kathryn E. Richards, M.D.
Clinical Assistant Professor of Surgery,
University of Michigan Medical Center
Co-Director of Michigan Burn Center

EMERGENT CARE OF THE BURN VICTIM

Published by the National Institute for Burn Medicine

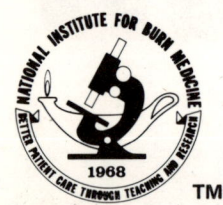

909 East Ann Street
Ann Arbor, Michigan 48104

ISBN 0-917478-49-5
Library of Congress Catalog Card number 75-15375

Copyright, 1977, by The National Institute for Burn Medicine

Copyright under the International Copyright Union. All Rights Reserved. This book is protected by Copyright. No part of it may be duplicated or reproduced in any manner without written permission of the publisher. Made in the United States of America.

Typesetting and layout — Sandra Kay Alexander

DEDICATION

to those emergency medical personnel who have assisted us in preparing this manual — and to those who will use it in the future.

PREFACE

First aid to the burn victim can make the difference between life and death and also reduce the severity of complications. Emergency medical workers (EMT's, firefighters, police, nurses, physicians, etc.) are in a position to make this difference.

The care of the burn patient is a team responsibility and it has only been within the last few years that the EMS workers and the Emergency Department personnel have been recognized as important members of the team. The objective of this manual is to provide the principles and practices necessary to improve the skills of the EMT and ED personnel as they become integrated into the team.

Burn care can be divided into three distinct but overlapping phases: the emergent, the acute, and the rehabilitative. The emergent phase begins at the time of the accident and continues until all lifesaving measures have been completed. This period may last anywhere from one to seven days or more. It is during this period of time that the immediate effects of the accident can be life-threatening. Care in the emergent period is lifesaving as well as preparatory for definitive therapy. Initial treatment given the severely burned patient at the scene of the accident and in the Emergency Department serves as the foundation on which continuing excellence of care is built.

The Emergent Care of the Burn Victim manual contains the information necessary to provide the care needed at the scene of the accident and in the Emergency Department. The manual is part of a "package" which also includes a film and an EMS burn care poster for use by all emergency care personnel. It is hoped that this teaching package will provide instructors as well as technicians and clinicians with the information and methodology necessary to improve the performance of emergency medical personnel.

TABLE OF CONTENTS

LIST OF FIGURES AND TABLES viii
ACKNOWLEDGEMENTS ix
FOREWORD xiii

I. INTRODUCTION TO THE BURN PROBLEM 1
   A. Incidence of Burn Accidents 1
   B. Etiology of Burns 1
      1. How? 1
      2. Who? 1
      3. Where? 2
   C. Anatomy and Physiology of the Skin 2
      1. Anatomy of the Skin 2
      2. Functions of the Skin 2
   D. Determining the Severity of the Burn 4
      1. Size of Burn 5
      2. Depth of Burn 6
      3. Differential Diagnosis of Depth of Burn 6
   E. First Aid in Burn Care 7

II. CARE AT THE SCENE OF THE ACCIDENT 9
   A. Initial Patient Survey 9
      1. Assess the Situation, Move Victim to Safety 9
      2. Initial Patient Contact 11
   B. Stop the Burning Process 12
      1. Thermal Injury (Flame, Hot-Surface, Sunburn) 12
      2. Scald Injury (Hot Water, Steam) 13
      3. Tar Burn 13
      4. Electrical or Lightning 13
      5. Chemical Injury 14
         a. Skin 14
         b. Eyes 15
      6. Frostbite 15
      7. Radiation 16
   C. First Aid for the Burned Victim: BREATHING, BLEEDING, SHOCK,
     Concurrent Injuries, and Severity of Burn 19
      1. Breathing: An Open AIRWAY is Essential to Survival 20
         a. Diagnosis 21
         b. Treatment 21
      2. Evaluate BLEEDING: Head to Toe Survey 22
         a. Diagnosis 22
         b. Treatment 22
      3. Shock: CIRCULATORY System Failure 22
         a. Diagnosis 23
         b. Treatment 23

D. Severity of the Burn 24
   1. Diagnosis 24
   2. Major Burn Wound Treatment 24
   3. Superficial Minor Burn Wound Treatment 25
E. Mass Casualties 25
F. Emotional Support 26
G. Transportation to the Emergency Department 27
H. Transition to Care in the Emergency Department 27

III. CARE OF THE VICTIM IN THE EMERGENCY DEPARTMENT 29
   A. First Aid in the Emergency Department 29
      1. Transition of Care 31
      2. Stop the Burning Process 31
         a. Thermal 31
         b. Chemical 32
         c. Tar 32
         d. Electrical 32
         e. Frostbite (see page 62) 32
         f. Radiation 34
      3. First Aid 36
         a. Airway (Immediate Respiratory Care) 36
         b. Bleeding 36
         c. Shock 37
         d. Concurrent Injuries 37
      4. Emotional Support 37
   B. Estimation of Severity of Injury 38
      1. Extent of Burn 38
      2. Depth of Burn 39
      3. Age 39
      4. Past Medical History 43
      5. Part of Body Burned and Concurrent Injuries 43
      6. Diagnosis of Minor or Major Burn 44
         a. Minor Burn 44
         b. Major Burn 44
         c. Level of Care Required 45
   C. Minor Burn Treatment in the Emergency Department 45
      1. Wound Care 46
      2. Comfort 46
      3. Infection 47
      4. Considerations for Outpatient Care 47
   D. Major Burn Care 48
      1. Respiratory Care 48
         a. Diagnosis 48
         b. Treatment 48
      2. Fluid Therapy 50
         a. Which Patients Require Fluid Therapy? 52
         b. Method of Fluid Therapy 52

       c. What Type of Fluids? ... 53
       d. How Much Fluid? ... 53
          1) Parameters of Therapy ... 53
          2) Output ... 55
          3) Physical Examination ... 56
          4) Hemoglobinuria ... 57
   3. Medications ... 57
       a. Infection Control ... 57
       b. Pain Relief ... 58
   4. Gastrointestinal Considerations ... 59
   5. Laboratory Testing ... 59
   6. Wound Care ... 59
       a. Immediate Transfer to Specialized Care ... 59
       b. Treatment in Non-Specialized Facility or Delay in Transfer ... 60
   7. Summary Charting ... 62
   8. Mass Casualties ... 62
 E. Frostbite (Rapid Thawing Treatment) ... 62
 F. Triage Considerations ... 64
   1. Explanation of Triage ... 64
   2. Decision to Triage (Where Should the Patient Be Treated?) ... 65
   3. Information to Give to Burn Care Facility Regarding Transfer of Patient ... 65
   4. Therapy Enroute to a Burn Care Facility ... 67
       a. Respiratory Support ... 67
       b. Fluid Therapy ... 67
       c. Urinary Output ... 68
       d. Gastrointestinal Support ... 68
       e. Wound Care ... 68
       f. Pain Relief ... 68
       g. Assess Condition ... 68
       h. Emotional Support ... 69
   5. Transition to Specialized Burn Care ... 69

IV. GLOSSARY OF TERMS ... 71

V. INDEX ... 75

LIST OF FIGURES AND TABLES

Figure	Title	Page
1	Anatomy of the Skin	3
2	Estimation of Size of Burn by Rule of Nines	5
3	Considerations for First Aid for the Burned Victim	8
4	EMS Burn Care Poster	30
5	Estimation of Size of Burn by Percent	40
6	Differential Diagnosis of Depth of Burn	41
7	Burn Patient Survival — Age Group vs Total Area Burned	42
8	Edema Formation	51
9	Example of Formulas for Fluid Therapy	54
10	Dressing Application	61
11	24 hour Summary Chart	63
12	Recommendations for Burn Care Facility Triage	66

Table	Title	Page
I	Functions of the Skin	3
II	Checklist for Care of Burned Victim at the Scene of the Accident	10
III	Definition of Minor and Major Burn	11
IV	Emergent Treatment of Chemical Burns	33

ACKNOWLEDGEMENTS

We wish to express special thanks to our colleagues and associates for their assistance in making this book possible.

CONTRIBUTORS: Mary E. Haab, R.N., Burn Nurse Specialist, Michigan Burn Center for general medical review; Jay S. Finch, M.D., Medical Director, Respiratory Therapy, Professor Anesthesiology, University of Michigan Medical Center for pulmonary management; Carl L. Pierson, Ph.D., Director Burn Center Laboratories, University of Michigan Burn Center for infection control; Eleanor Strang, R.N., Director of Nursing Service, Holver Medical Center, Gallipolis Ohio for initial data gathering; John H. Van de Leuv, M.D., C.M., Director of Emergency Department, Coordinator, EMT Training Program, Wyandotte General Hospital for meticulous attention to medical editing of the manuscript; John W. Keyes, Jr., M.D., Associate Professor of Internal Medicine and Radiology, University of Michigan Medical Center; James E. Carey, M.S., Assistant Professor of Radiation Physics, Internal Medicine, University of Michigan Medical Center, R.F. Rentenbach, M.D., Detroit Edison Company, and Arthur J. Solari, Director, Radiation Control Service, University of Michigan for section on Radiation Therapy; James R. Lloyd, M.D., Director of Burn Care, Children's Hospital of Michigan, Detroit, for suggestions on care of burned children, and Janise J. Mac Kichan, Pharm.D., Pharmacy Department, University of Michigan Medical Center for review of Table on Emergent Treatment of Chemical Burns.

ASSISTANCE IN MANUSCRIPT COMPLETION: Cynthia Wojtowicz, Administrator, and Michael H. James, Director of Program Development, National Institute for Burn Medicine for administrative assistance, Mary K. Bailey, Eleanor Dill, and Karen Gilson for deciphering and typing numerous manuscripts; James E. Haney for editing; Julia Casa, Librarian, National Institute for Burn Medicine for library assistance, Sam Flanders for statistical analysis; and Mary K. Bailey for indexing.

FINANCIAL ASSISTANCE OF THE EMS BURN INFORMATION AND TRIAGE SYSTEM: The W.K. Kellogg Great Lakes Regional Burn Care Development Program, the Michigan Association for Regional Medical Programs and an Innovation and Expansion Grant from the Michigan Department of Education, Vocational Rehabilitation Service.

MEDICAL REVIEW OF MANUSCRIPT: Syed Akhtar, M.D., Director of Burn Care, St. Mary's Hospital, Saginaw; Robert Aranosian, D.O., Director of Emergency Department, Pontiac Osteopathic Hospital; Gene R. Arindaeng, M.D., Director of Emergency Department, Metropolitan Hospital, Detroit; Rebecca S. Cole, EMS Associate, East Michigan EMS; Charles F. Frey, M.D., Professor and Vice Chairman, Department of Surgery, University of California at Davis; Harry Hayden; Martin L. Jackier, M.D., Chief, Emergency Care Services Section, Macomb Hospital Association, Detroit; Catherine Janice, R.N., Associate Director, Ambulatory Services, Harper-Grace Hospitals, Detroit; Patrick W. LaFleur, D.O., Director, Emergency Department, Detroit Osteopathic Hospitals, Highland Park; Mark Nelson; Frank Newman, M.D., Director of Burn Care, Bronson Hospital, Kalamazoo; Melva Parks, R.N., Director, Emergency Department, McNamara Community Hospital, Warren; Aldean Reynolds, Director of Inservice Education, Saratoga General Hospital, Detroit; and Sid Smock, M.D., Director of Emergency Department Services, St. Mary's Hospital, Livonia.

EMERGENT CARE OF THE BURN VICTIM 　　　　　　　　　　　　　　　　　**National Institute for Burn Medicine**

ASSISTANCE BY THE SOUTHEASTERN MICHIGAN REGIONAL TASK FORCE ON EMERGENCY MEDICAL SERVICES FOR EMS REVIEW OF MANUSCRIPT: Michigan Department of Public Health, Division of Emergency Medical Services; Ronald L. Krome, M.D., Chairman, Southeastern Michigan Regional Task Force on Emergency Medical Services; Dale D. Pelton, Senior Health Planner, Comprehensive Health Planning Council of Southeastern Michigan, and the County Health Department EMS Coordinators: Beth Beekman, Livingston County; Dick Buss, Wayne County; Gary Canfield, Oakland County; Mary Kay Mastracci and Jan Szandzik, Macomb County; Ken Montgomery, St. Clair County; Richard Muhs, Washtenaw County; Lou Watling, Monroe County, and the following:

- **Emergency Departments**

Livingston County

McPherson Community Health Center
Howell

Macomb County

Harrison Community Hospital
Mt. Clemens

Mt. Clemens General Hospital

St. Joseph Hospital
Mt. Clemens

Bi-County Community Hospital
Warren

McNamara Community Hospital of Warren

Memorial Hospital of Warren

South Macomb Hospital
Warren

Monroe County

Memorial Hospital of Monroe

Mercy Hospital of Monroe

Oakland County

Madison Community Hospital

Martin Place Hospital
Madison Heights

Pontiac General Hospital

Pontiac Osteopathic Hospital

St. Joseph Mercy Hospital

Crittenton Hospital
Rochester

William Beaumont Hospital
Royal Oak

Providence Hospital
Southfield

St. Clair County

Mercy Hospital
Port Huron

Port Huron Hospital

River District Hospital
St. Clair

Yale Community Hospital

Washtenaw County

St. Joseph Mercy Hospital
Ann Arbor

University Hospital
Ann Arbor

Chelsea Community Hospital

Saline Community Hospital

Beyer Memorial Hospital
Ypsilanti

Wayne County

Oakwood Hospital
Dearborn

Art Centre Hospital
Detroit

Children's Hospital
Detroit

Detroit General Hospital

Detroit Memorial Hospital

Evangelical Deaconess Hospital
Detroit

Grace Hospital, N.W.
Detroit

Harper Hospital
Detroit

Henry Ford Hospital
Detroit

Holy Cross Hospital
Detroit

Hutzel Hospital
Detroit

Lakeside Medical Center
Detroit

Martin Place — West
Detroit

Metropolitan Hospital
Detroit

Mount Carmel Mercy Hospital
Detroit

North Detroit General Hospital

Plymouth General Hospital
Detroit

Redford Community Hospital
Detroit

St. John's Hospital
Detroit

St. Joseph's Mercy Hospital
Detroit

Saratoga General Hospital
Detroit

Sinai Hospital of Detroit

Southwest Detroit Hospital

Ziegler Osteopathic Hospital
Detroit

Wayne County General Hospital
Eloise

Botsford General Hospital
Farmington

Garden City Osteopathic Hospital

Bon Secours Hospital
Grosse Pointe

Cottage Hospital of Grosse Pointe

Detroit Osteopathic Hospital
Highland Park

Lynn Hospital
Lincoln Park

Outer Drive Hospital
Lincoln Park

St. Mary's Hospital
Livonia

Sidney A. Sumby Memorial Hospital
River Rouge

Seaway Hospital
Trenton

National Institute for Burn Medicine — EMERGENT CARE OF THE BURN VICTIM

Emergency Departments (cont.)

Annapolis Hospital
Wayne

Metropolitan Hospital — West
Westland

Wyandotte General Hospital

- **Private/Public Ambulance Services:**

Meda Care Ambulance Company
Dearborn

All Saints Ambulance
Detroit

Alpha Community Development Corporation
Detroit

Ambro Ambulance
Detroit

Detroit Fire Department
EMS Division

Michigan Ambulance Inc.
Detroit

Shuttle Ambulance Service
Detroit

Farmington Hills Ambulance Service
Farmington Hills

Huron Valley Ambulance
Highland Twp.

Holly Volunteer Ambulance, Inc.

Novi Ambulance Service

Sherman Ambulance Service
Ortonville

Fleet Ambulance Service, Inc.
Pontiac

Northland Ambulance Service
Pontiac

Riverside Chapel Ambulance Service
Pontiac

St. Onge Ambulance Corporation
Rochester

Suburban Ambulance Service, Inc.
Royal Oak

County Ambulance Service, Inc.
Southfield

Taylor Ambulance Service
Taylor

- **Municipal Fire Departments:**

Ann Arbor Fire Department

Berkely Fire Department

Birmingham Fire Department

Dearborn Fire Department

Dearborn Heights Fire Department

Detroit Fire Department, Fire Fighting Division

East Detroit Fire Department

Farmington Hills Fire Department

Ferndale Fire Department

Garden City Fire Department

Harrison Township Fire Department

Hazel Park Fire Department

Addison Twp. Fire Department
Leonard

Livonia Fire Department

Madison Heights Fire Department

Mt. Clemens Fire Department

Oak Park Public Safety Department

Pontiac Fire Department

Wayne County Detroit Metropolitan Airport Fire Department
Romulus

Southfield Fire Department

Southgate Fire Department

South Lyon Fire Department

Sterling Heights Fire Department

Taylor Fire Department

Shelby Twp. Fire Department
Utica

Warren Fire Department

Wayne Fire Department

Westland Fire Department

- **College EMT Training Programs:**

Oakland County Community College
Auburn Heights
Dick Osgoode

Monroe County Community College
Monroe
Bob Neville

Henry Ford Community College
Dearborn
Dorothy Caponi

Kalamazoo Valley Community College
Kalamazoo
Michael La Penera

Kellogg Community College
Battle Creek
Tom Klopfenstein

Lansing Community College
Lansing
Rexine Finn

Macomb County Community College
Mt. Clemens
Sam Petros

Madonna College
Livonia
Diane Krzston

Mercy College of Detroit
Detroit
David Ballinger

Mid Michigan Community College
Harrison
Robert L. Klute

Mott Community College
Flint
James Parcerelli

Muskegan Community College
Muskegan
Robert Nelson

North Central Michigan College
Petoskey
Arthur Frances

St. Clair County Community College
Port Huron
Clarence Knight

Southwestern Michigan Community College
Dowagiac
Westley Z. Muth

Washtenaw Community College
Ann Arbor
Scott Turik

Wayne County Community College
Detroit
Mary Hunt

FOREWORD

The emergent care of the burned victim presents some of the most challenging and demanding problems to be encountered in the whole spectrum of human injury. The development of a well-coordinated team effort, which draws upon the expertise of multiple specialists in Medicine, Nursing and Allied Health Professions, is strategically important to a successful outcome. The authors of this timely manual have long recognized this need. They have been instrumental nationally in establishing channels of communication with, and in securing the participatory involvement of, a host of different emergency medical workers in attempting to resolve the many problems presented by the burned victim.

Their previous publication <u>Nursing the Burned Patient</u> (1973) focused successfully upon the essential role which the nursing profession plays in this team effort. This manual is directed primarily to that highly important first echelon of the Burn Team, the Emergency Medical Technician who serves in the ambulance or Emergency Department. Although written in direct and readily understandable prose, it summarizes effectively the authors' wide clinical experience, productive research, and statistical analyses in Burn Medicine. It should prove to be an invaluable guide and source of information, not only to the EMT, and Emergency Department physicians and nurses, but to countless numbers of other professionals as well — firefighters, police, nursing students, medical students and hospital house officers among them.

Finally, the authors present a provocative blueprint for the regionalization of care of the critically burned patient. The various and progressive responsibilities of the EMT are clearly outlined for each phase of burn treatment as the patient passes along the therapeutic network from the site of injury to the highly sophisticated Burn Center — every move is graphically described or diagrammed. Those observations or corrective measures which may be life saving are emphasized — and re-emphasized. Nothing is left to chance if it can be anticipated and programmed. Therein lies the secret of successful Burn Management — and of the authors' pre-eminence in this field.

M.S. DeWeese, M.D., F.A.C.S.
Clinical Professor of Surgery
University of Michigan

INTRODUCTION TO THE BURN PROBLEM

Incidence of Burn Accidents

Burns are the third largest cause of accidental death in the United States, exceeded only by motor vehicle accidents and falls. In the age group 0 to 5 years, fires and burns are the leading cause of death. Nearly 2,200,000 people are burned badly enough to seek medical attention each year; of these 75,000 are hospitalized, and 9,000 die from their burns. In Michigan, approximately 100,000 are burned each year and of these 3,200 are hospitalized.

Etiology of Burns: How?, Who?, Where?

How? Burn injuries are caused by heat from flame, hot liquids, or hot surfaces; by electrical currents; by chemicals; or by radiation. Extreme cold, producing frostbite or freezing, causes an injury requiring treatment similar to the burn injury. Flame (fire) causes two-thirds of all burn injuries. The second-largest cause of burn injuries are scalds or contact with a hot surface. Next are chemical and radiation burns. Note particularly that *85% of all flame burns involve ignition of fabrics.* If clothing catches fire, the injury, length of hospital stay, and hospital costs increase dramatically.

If clothing ignites the severity of injury is greatly increased.

Who? Burn victims fall into five categories. In the largest category, 70%, are those who are victims of their own action, e.g., the child whose clothing ignites while playing with matches. 20% are innocent bystanders, such as the person burned at home by a furnace explosion. In the third category

---

All National Burn Information Exchange etiology statistics given here are taken from a data gathering and analysis project specific to burns sponsored by the National Institute for Burn Medicine. Planning and Designing a Burn Care Facility; Feller, Crane; Ann Arbor, Michigan; National Institute for Burn Medicine, 1971 lists these statistics.

are the 4% with a medical condition that predisposes them to the accident: for example, the epileptic person injured during a seizure. Intended victims make up another 4%, typified by the child intentionally burned by a parent as punishment. Rescue workers, such as the fireman injured in the line of duty, form the final category, comprising only 1% of the total. Even though these workers frequently risk contact with flame and possible burn, few are injured, due largely to effective safety precautions.

Due to effective safety precautions the incidence of rescue workers burned is decreased.

Different age groups sustain different types of burn injuries. Among toddlers, scalds are more common than flame burns. Industrial burns involving caustic elements or hot liquids are more common in adult males. Flame burns are frequently sustained by children playing with matches who set themselves or the building in which they are playing on fire. Infants and small children are also more susceptible to sunburn.

In the last ten years an alarming increase in inflicted burns to children has been noted. It is important to recognize and report any suspected neglect or intended injury so that the situation may be adequately evaluated. Failure to recognize a particular home or environmental situation as hazardous may permit a child to return to a potentially lethal home.

Where? 85% of all burn injuries occur in the home, while 15% occur either at work or in recreational areas. The kitchen, the bathroom, and the bedroom (in that order) are rooms most often involved in home accidents.

85% of all burns occur at home.

C. **Anatomy and Physiology of the Burned Organ, the Skin**

1. **Anatomy of the Skin**

The skin is the largest organ of the body (1.8 square meters or about 2 square yards, in the adult male), providing much more than a tough, pliable surface covering. It has two anatomic layers called the epidermis and the dermis (Figure 1). The epidermis, the outer nonvascular layer, is very thin and consists of layers of epithelial cells which, as they mature, form a protective covering of dead cells. The thicker dermis makes up the bulk of the skin. Its thickness ranges from 0.02 inch on the eyelid to 0.24 inch on the back. The skin serves as a physical barrier against hazards of the environment, such as infection.

The skin is the largest organ of the body.

2. **Functions of the Skin**

The skin has many functions (Table 1). One of the

National Institute for Burn Medicine   EMERGENT CARE OF THE BURN VICTIM

FIGURE 1

ANATOMY OF THE SKIN

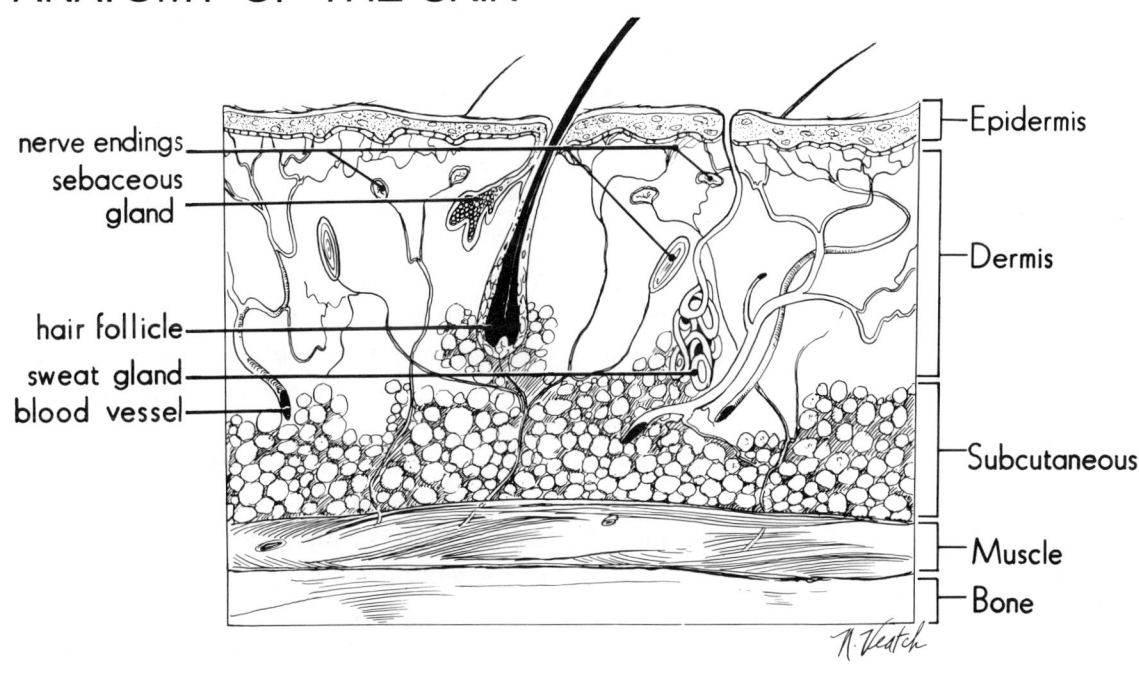

TABLE 1

FUNCTIONS OF THE SKIN

1. PROTECTS AGAINST INFECTION
2. PREVENTS LOSS OF BODY FLUIDS
3. CONTROLS BODY TEMPERATURE
4. EXCRETES SOME WASTE PRODUCTS
5. RECEIVES SENSORY STIMULI
6. PRODUCES VITAMIN D
7. DETERMINES IDENTITY (e.g., COSMETIC)

EMERGENT CARE OF THE BURN VICTIM

National Institute for Burn Medicine

The two most important functions of the skin are protection against infection and preservation of body fluids.

most important is protection against infection by maintaining a physical barrier to keep out bacteria and other organisms. The structure of the skin also prevents loss of body fluids, a function essential to avoiding dehydration and maintaining the delicate fluid balance required by the body.

Body temperature is controlled by the increasing or decreasing evaporation of water from the sweat glands. The sweat glands excrete excess water and small amounts of sodium chloride, cholestorin, traces of albumin and urea.

The skin is an extensive sensory organ. Nerve endings located within the dermis convey impulses which indicate whether a stimulus is light touch, pressure, pain, hot, or cold, thus allowing us to modify our immediate environment to avoid damage or destruction.

The sebacious glands protect the skin by secretion of oils which soften and lubricate. Vitamin D is made within the skin when sunlight reacts with cholesterol compounds.

The cosmetic effect of the skin varies from individual to individual and serves not only to identify by color but also by the various individual textures of skin, such as the whorls and patterns of fingerprints.

When the skin is burned, these functions are either diminished (when there is a partial-thickness burn) or eliminated (when there is complete destruction of the skin). Burn severity is determined to a great extent by the amount of skin lost, and the depth of the damage. Trauma results in decreased function or complete loss of the two most important life-preserving functions of the skin: protection against infection, and prevention of loss of body fluids. However, once the patient has recovered these functions, the loss of cosmetic appearance and pleasure-pain sensations may complicate the patient's readjustment to society.

D. <u>Determining the Severity of the Burn</u>

All burns are not alike. Severity is influenced by size and depth of the burn, age, past medical history and parts of the body injured.

All burns are not alike. Severity is influenced by five main factors: (1) size of burn; (2) depth of burn; (3) age; (4) past medical history; and (5) part of the body injured and concurrent injuries.

These factors are considered in combination when evaluating severity. However, for the purpose of explanation, each will be discussed separately.

National Institute for Burn Medicine   **EMERGENT CARE OF THE BURN VICTIM**

1. Size of Burn

The size of the burn is expressed as a percent of the total body area. There are two basic methods to determine this size. The first method, termed the *Rule of Nines,* is in frequent use because it is simple and quick, but unless diagrams are used it is not totally accurate. The head and each entire upper extremity (shoulder to fingertips, glove-fashion) are *each* given the value of 9% of the body surface. The anterior and posterior trunk are each valued at 18%, as is each leg. The total of these parts is 99% and the perineum is valued at 1% to make 100%. This method may be used visually at the scene of the accident to quickly estimate the size of burn. When the area of burn on the patient is shaded in on the drawing, one can determine a more accurate size of the burn. Use of the Rule of Nines to illustrate a 36% burn is shown in Figure 2. (The palm of the hand represents about 1% total body area; use of this fact may assist in estimation.)

The palm of the hand equals about 1% of the body.

FIGURE 2

ESTIMATION OF SIZE OF BURN BY RULE OF NINES

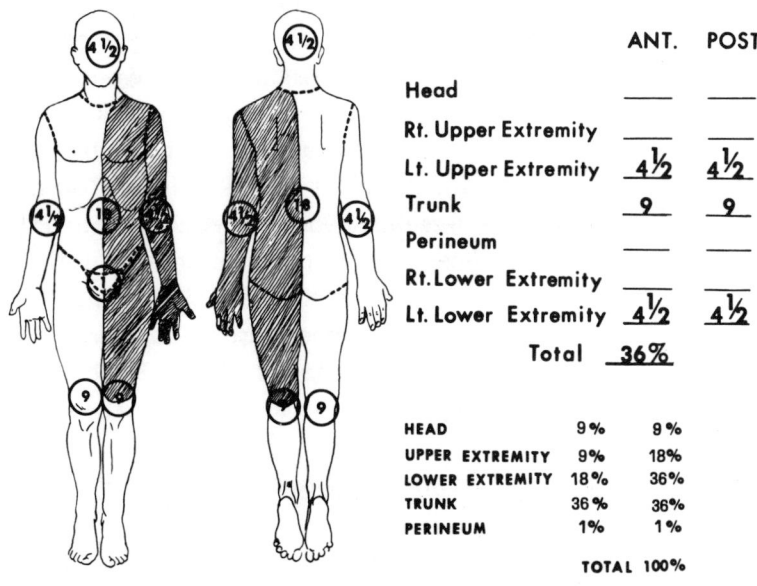

	ANT.	POST.
Head	——	——
Rt. Upper Extremity	——	——
Lt. Upper Extremity	4½	4½
Trunk	9	9
Perineum	——	——
Rt. Lower Extremity	——	——
Lt. Lower Extremity	4½	4½
Total	36%	

HEAD	9%	9%
UPPER EXTREMITY	9%	18%
LOWER EXTREMITY	18%	36%
TRUNK	36%	36%
PERINEUM	1%	1%
	TOTAL	100%

ADVANTAGES

1. Easily Done Without Use of Table

DISADVANTAGES

1. Inaccurate
2. Does Not Allow for Differences in Proportion of Head and Lower Extremities in Infants and Children as Compared to Adults

The second method requires figures and tables, and is more accurate, because it takes into account the change in proportion by age, of the head and lower extremities. This method is explained in the section on Emergency Department Care. (See Figure 5.)

2. **Depth of Burn**

Depth of burn is expressed as full-thickness or partial-thickness.

The depth of a burn is expressed in terms of full-thickness or partial-thickness. The classification of burns into "first," "second," and "third" degrees attempts to describe the depth of tissue damage, but these terms are not really descriptive of the injury, and give only visual characteristics of the wound. We now prefer the classification of partial- or full-thickness burn. The term partial-thickness burn means that only part of the skin has been damaged or destroyed. Enough epithelial cells remain in hair follicles and sweat glands to grow new skin. This wound will heal by itself if nothing in treatment causes further damage. The partial-thickness burn is equivalent to the first- or second-degree burn.

Full-thickness skin loss cannot heal by itself, it must be grafted.

Full-thickness burns are defined as those where all of the skin is destroyed and possibly subcutaneous tissue, muscle, and bone, depending upon temperature and duration of exposure to the burning agent. Regeneration of the skin is not possible. These wounds must be grafted to provide cover and return normal skin function. They are serious wounds because the body has lost the life-preserving functions of the skin in the burned area. A full-thickness burn wound is equivalent to a third-degree burn. The deeper the burn, the more serious the problem.

With good care, partial-thickness injury can reheal.

The skin of the small child is slightly thinner than the adult and a similar insult (compared to an adult) may result in a more severe injury. The basic principles of evaluation of depth, however, remain the same.

3. **Differential Diagnosis of Depth of Burn**

The depth of burn is difficult to determine visually. There are signs and symptoms which indicate the level of tissue damaged, but the exact depth of injury can be determined only when spontaneous healing has taken place or granulation tissue has appeared after eschar removal.

Estimating the depth of burn immediately after the accident is of little value to emergency care. However, because depth of injury is considered in triage, Figure 6 describes differential diagnosis of depth. (Triage refers to the system of determining the severity of the burn and transferring the victim to the level of specialized care necessary to optimally meet his needs.)

The other severity factors (age, past medical history, part of body burned, and concurrent injuries) are discussed in the section of this book on Care in the Emergency Room.

E. <u>First Aid in Burn Care</u>

Care of the burned victim can be divided into systemic care and local care. Systemic care includes measures that maintain function of the various organ systems—heart, lung, kidneys, etc.—to maintain life. Throughout history, until World War II, treatment of the burn injury was primarily local—merely wound care—and because of this patients died needlessly. This concern for wound care and lack of attention to systemic care can be explained by the obvious and usually unsightly wound. Mortality of burn victims, however, has decreased in the last 20 years. We now recognize the burn victim as a trauma victim requiring immediate *systemic* treatment.

When the burn is major, emphasis is on systemic treatment. This does not mean, though, that wound care is unimportant or can be neglected. The ABC's of first aid, concerning **BREATHING, BLEEDING,** and **SHOCK,** come before wound care. Wound care is essential to survival, but may be delayed for a few hours until all life-saving measures have been taken.

There are three levels of first aid for the burned individual. The first is at the scene of the accident, the second is in the Emergency Department, and the third is in a specialized burn care facility (Figure 3). The *principles* of first aid remain the same throughout these phases; only the *intensity* of care differs. Through this repetition of first aid, even the most severely burned victim is given a better chance for survival.

The burn victim is a trauma victim requiring immediate first aid.

FIGURE 3

CONSIDERATIONS FOR FIRST AID OF THE BURN VICTIM

		Scene of Accident	Emergency Department	Burn Care Facility
1.	Stop the Burning Process	✓	✓	✓
2.	Provide an Open Airway	✓	✓	✓
3.	Stop Bleeding	✓	✓	✓
4.	Prevent Shock	✓	✓	✓
5.	Treat Concurrent Injuries	✓	✓	✓
6.	Care for the Wound	✓	✓	✓
7.	Provide Emotional Support	✓	✓	✓
8.	Transport the Patient	✓	✓	

II. CARE AT THE SCENE OF THE ACCIDENT

Decisive and immediate care for the burn victim at the scene of the accident can make the difference between life and death. The EMT arriving at the scene of the accident should be able to (1) assess the situation quickly but thoroughly, identifying the victim(s), entry to the victim(s), and possible hazards for the victim(s), the EMT(s), and bystanders; and (2) immediately stop the burning process, assess the severity of the injury, and provide necessary treatment.

The well-trained emergency medical worker develops a mental checklist (refer to Table II). *Assessment and treatment for one victim should usually take no longer than 15 minutes.* That is, the patient should receive immediate care and be on the way to the Emergency Department in this time. Proper immediate attention and rapid transport are vital. Wound care involves only prevention of further trauma. Definitive therapy begins in the Emergency Department or specialized care facility.

The well-trained EMT has a mental checklist for immediate assessment and treatment.

Table III details the difference between a minor and major burn. All those in the major burn category require medical attention. The rule is to transport all major and minor burns to the Emergency Department for evaluation.

Respiratory distress may not be immediately obvious; however, there are clearcut indicators of impending distress. Burn wound care is not life-saving at the scene of the accident. Systemic care takes precedence.

A. Initial Patient Survey

1. Assess the Situation and Move Victim to Safety

Upon arrival at the scene of the accident, the EMT does not always find an already identified victim lying in a safe place waiting for first aid. Burn accident victims should be conscious and able to talk rationally. However, due to the accident, many behave irrationally. Frequently the emergency medical worker will be called on to assess the situation and decide on the appropriate methods of

Move the victim to safety.

EMERGENT CARE OF THE BURN VICTIM   National Institute for Burn Medicine

TABLE II

CHECKLIST FOR CARE OF THE BURNED VICTIM AT THE SCENE OF THE ACCIDENT

1. **Assess the Accident Scene for:**

   - location of victims(s).
   - best access to victim(s).
   - possible hazard to victim(s), EMT(s), and bystander(s).

2. **Stop the Burning Process:**

   - roll victim on ground.
   - smother flames with blanket.
   - use low-pressure water.

3. **Move the Victim(s) to Safety.**

4. **Complete the Initial Patient Survey:**

   - speak to victim:

     → determine the level of consciousness. (A burn does not render the victim unconscious, he should be conscious and able to talk to you.)
     → can the patient talk to you, respond to pain, move body parts?
     → acknowledge his/her primary injury.

   - determine possible respiratory involvement:

     → burned in enclosed space (forced to breath smoke)?
     → soot in nose or mouth?
     → face burn?
     → difficult respirations?

   - provide an open airway and high concentration of oxygen.
   - check vital signs: blood pressure, pulse, respiration.
   - does the victim have a stiff or sore neck (possible cervical injury)?
   - examine the total body:

     → cut away clothes on injured areas.
     → estimate percent of burn (Rule of Nines).
     → check for fractures, lacerations, concurrent injuries.

5. **Treat Concurrent Injury According to Accepted Practice.**

6. **Care for the Wound: Wrap in Clean, Dry, or Sterile Sheet and Cover with Blanket for Warmth.**

7. **Provide Emotional Support.**

8. **Transport to the Appropriate Emergency Department or Facility.**

NOTE: The victim should have received all of the above care at the scene of the accident and be enroute to an Emergency Department within 15 minutes. Each of these steps is discussed in detail on the following pages.

National Institute for Burn Medicine EMERGENT CARE OF THE BURN VICTIM

TABLE III

MINOR AND MAJOR BURN DEFINITION

Minor Burn

It is a *minor* burn if:

- The injury is less than 10% of the total body area.
- The patient is less than 35 years old.
- The patient is more than 4 years old.
- The medical history is negative for chronic and severe illnesses.
- The burn does not include the face, hands, feet, perineum, and is not circumferential.
- There are no significant concurrent injuries (i.e., respiratory damage, fracture, etc.).
- It is not an electrical injury.
- Individual considerations (i.e., patient capable of managing own outpatient care).

Major Burn

It is a *major* burn if:

- The injury is greater than 10% of the total body area.
- The patient is more than 35 years old.
- The patient is less than 4 years old.
- The medical history shows chronic or severe illnesses.
- There are burns of the face, hands, feet, perineum, or there are circumferential burns.
- There are significant concurrent injuries (i.e., respiratory damage, fracture, etc.).
- The victim cannot manage home care or is suspected of sustaining physical abuse.

---

rescue and treatment. To the experienced worker this may be second nature. To the novice this may be a difficult aspect of care. The first task is to locate the victim or victims, establish access to them, and identify environmental hazards (such as electrical current, explosive gases, etc.) to the victim, rescuer, and bystanders. The victim(s) must then be moved to safety. Some find the burned victim unsightly and are put off by the appearance of the wound. Burned tissue will not be further damaged by gentle handling. Common sense and standard rescue techniques should dictate precautions in moving the victim.

Burned tissue will NOT be further damaged by gentle handling.

2. **Initial Patient Contact**

Once the victim(s) has been identified, the EMT should introduce him/her self to the victim. This is not only courtesy;—this simple act announces to the victim that help has arrived—step one in providing emotional support. More importantly, it allows the rescuer to determine the victim's level of consciousness. The victim should be able to talk—*a burn injury does not render the victim unconscious, even a burn of 100% total body area.* If the victim cannot speak or speak coherently, immediately look for a cause other than the burn: anoxia from prolonged inhalation of noxious (poisonous) fumes, stroke, heart attack, head injury, etc. Give oxygen as soon as possible.

A burn injury does NOT render the victim unconscious! Look for another cause.

During the initial conversation *acknowledge the victims primary injury.* For instance, if the hands are burned the victim may say, "My hands are burned, they hurt." The EMT replies, "Yes, I see your hands are burned. I am here to take care of you." This recognition of the victim's concern is a second step to provide emotional support. It is important to know that *emotional support* is not a procedure to be taught; it is a genuine concern for the well-being of the patient. The patient will feel confidence if you are able to communicate concern, interest, and a feeling that things are now under control.

Acknowledge the victim's primary complaint.

B. Stop the Burning Process

The intensity of the heat (or burning agent) and length of time of contact with the skin determines the depth and extent of injury (refer to Figure 6). The first step in treating any burn victim is to *stop the burning process* and reduce penetration of the burning agent into deeper tissues. Use the quickest, most convenient extinguishing means available for stopping the burning process. Roll the victim on the ground, use a blanket and smother flames, use low-pressure water if available. Ice treatment is not recommended, because extreme cold can further traumatize already damaged tissue. Cool water is preferred to reduce the penetration of heat into deeper tissue.

STOP the burning process.

Extreme cold — ice water — can further traumatize damaged tissue.

1. Thermal Injury (Flame, Hot-Surface, Sunburn)

Objective: To remove the heat source and to reduce the penetration of heat into deeper tissue.

- Roll the victim on the ground.
- Spray water on the burning individual. If a water hose is used, **use low pressure.**
- Smother the flames with a non-flammable blanket, coat, or other heavy fabric.
- Immerse the burned area in cool water.

- Once the heat source is removed, check for and extinguish smoldering or steaming clothing. Use scissors to remove any clothing which will retain heat. Do not, however, remove or peel clothing which has adhered to the wound.

Remove clothing which may hold heat.

2. **Scald Injury (Hot Water and Steam)**

   Objective: To reduce the penetration of heat to deep tissues.

   - Remove clothing which may hold heat.
   - Immerse the scalded area in *cool* water for a few minutes.
     (Note: cool water is effective only if used within a few minutes after the accident.)
   - Do not break blisters.

3. **Tar Burns**

   Objective: To remove the coating of hot tar, reduce penetration of heat to deeper tissues, and protect the underlying burned skin.

   Hot tar causing the burn leaves a coating of tar on the wound that is best removed by immediate immersion of the wound in ice water. This dissipates the heat, hardens the tar, and causes it to shrink away from the skin. Do not attempt to remove the tar. Transport the victim to special care as soon as possible.

   Immerse tar-coated wound in ice water. The ice water will harden the tar for removal.

   - Immerse and soak the tar-coated area in ice water or very cool water (2 to 3 minutes).
   - Remove area from the ice water.
   - Do not attempt to remove the tar if it does not peel away easily. (Immerse in ice water again.)
   - If tar cannot be rapidly cooled for removal, do not attempt to peel the tar from the wound.
   - Elevate the head if the tar burn is of the face and/or neck. Elevation of tar burns of the extremities also reduces swelling.

4. **Electrical or Lightning Injuries**

   Objective: To remove the victim from the electrical current.

   The most common immediate problem from an

EMERGENT CARE OF THE BURN VICTIM National Institute for Burn Medicine

Cardio-pulmonary arrest is the most common immediate problem in electrical or lightning injury.

An electrical (or lightning) injury will result in an entry and exit wound, as well as thermal injury if clothing ignites.

For chemical burn, flood the tissue with water to totally remove the chemical.

electrical or lightning accident is cardio-pulmonary arrest. Rapid resuscitation is needed. An entry and exit wound usually result from electrical or lightning injuries, but very little immediate attention to these wounds is required at the scene of the accident. The primary concern is to stop the electrical current and prevent or treat cardio-pulmonary arrest.

The entry and exit wound usually appear small on the surface (coin-size) unless there was also clothing ignition. These wounds require hospitalization for observation and/or treatment regardless of size.

- Remove the electrical source. *The rescuer must take all precautions not to contact the electrical source or the victim while he/she is in contact with the electrical source.* (Follow recommended EMS procedure for removing electrical source.)
- If the electrical source ignited clothing, see Thermal Injury (No. 1) above.
- Perform cardio-pulmonary resuscitation (CPR) as necessary.

5. **Chemical Injury**

Objective: To remove the burning agent and reduce penetration into deeper tissues.

In most chemical injuries, the first step is to dilute the chemical with large amounts of water. A few chemicals may react with water to form a greater irritant. However, because rescuers and EMT's do not routinely carry neutralizers, and because any neutralization agent may also generate additional heat, authorities recommend copious water flooding for *all* chemical burns. When using water lavage, *always* completely flood the area with water to totally eliminate the chemical.

a. <u>Skin</u>

- Remove any clothing that may hold the chemical in contact with the skin.
- Flush the burned area immediately with *great volumes* of cool water.
- Continue to flood the skin as clothing is being removed.
- Clothing soaked with gasoline (kerosine, cleaning fluids, and other volatile solutions) should be totally water flooded and removed to prevent the

possibility of further ignition.
- If at all possible, identify the type of chemical so that if further neutralization and/or treatment is necessary, it may be done in the Emergency Department.
- Refer to Table IV for more details on treatment of chemical burns.

b. **Eyes**

- Flush gently with copious amounts of cool, clean water. You cannot use too much water to flush the eyes. *Use low pressure; do not use water under high pressure.*
- Carefully lift the upper and lower lids to allow thorough flushing.
  CAUTION: The chemical may react with small amounts of water to form a greater irritant. Therefore, **the chemical must be completely eliminated by flooding with water.**

Use low pressure water to flood chemical burn of the eyes.

6. **Frostbite**

Objective: To remove the victim from the cold and to reintroduce warmth to the tissues without causing additional trauma.

Cold injuries may be divided into three categories: (1) non-freezing, (2) frostbite, and (3) total body cooling.

Non-freezing injuries of the immersion or "trench foot" type are most commonly seen in wartime and result from exposure to cold temperatures for many hours or days, resulting in an injury noted for extensive edema, pain, and slow recovery.

Acute freezing injury, properly designated *frostbite*, is more commonly a civilian injury due to a brief acute exposure to subfreezing temperatures. Prior to thawing the part is hard, cold, usually white, or yellowish-white, and anesthetic. The part appears to be solidly frozen even in partial-thickness injury.

A third category is *total body cooling* (hypothermia) from prolonged or severe exposure to freezing temperatures. Once body temperature drops below 94° to 88°F, depression, coma, cardio-pulmonary failure, and death may follow.

When confronted by a cold injury, the primary consideration, as with all trauma victims, is basic first aid.

The primary consideration for the frostbite victim is first aid.

EMERGENT CARE OF THE BURN VICTIM National Institute for Burn Medicine

Extremes of heat or cold will only further damage frozen tissue.

Once the cardio-pulmonary and central nervous systems have been evaluated and treated, attention is turned to the wound. Under NO circumstances should the injured area be chaffed with snow or immersed in ice water, even though this is less painful, *or* exposed to temperatures over 106°F. The frozen tissue is already damaged and extremes of heat and cold can *only* add more damage.

Remove the victim from the cold as rapidly as possible. If absolutely necessary, he/she may walk on frozen legs and feet to escape the cold. However, if the legs and feet have thawed, carry the victim. Above all, protect the injured area from further trauma.

- Provide basic first aid; an open airway, stop bleeding, control shock.
- Treat for concurrent trauma (e.g., fracture).
- Remove the victim from the cold.
- *Wrap the body or injured part in warm blankets.* (Remember the frozen body part can generate no heat.)
  - *Do not* allow the victim to walk on the thawed part.
  - *Do not* place hot (over 106° F) water or packs on the injured areas.
  - *Do not* massage or rub the injured area.
- Do not break blisters or remove tissue from the wound.
- Transport to Emergency Department immediately.

7. **Radiation Burns**

Objective: To provide life-sustaining treatment to the victim of radiation injury.

Although the use of nuclear energy has greatly increased, serious radiation accidents continue to be infrequent. This record can be attributed to the work of radiation safety experts and competent performance. Radiation injury does not provide an immediate "burn wound" per se. Immediate trauma to the victim will more likely be in the form of associated injury. Care at the scene is the same as for other trauma victims; the hazard, if any, lies in rescuing the victim from the radiation source while reducing the amount of exposure to possibly harmful rays and particles for the rescuer and bystanders. **There is no recorded instance that anyone received an intolerable dose of radiation while caring for a radiation accident victim during first aid or in the hospital.**

Radiation injury can result in a local or systemic

response or both. The injuries which may be seen involving radiation are (a) "burns" from radiation exposure, but *no* contamination; (b) "burns" from radiation exposure plus contamination; and (c) thermally and/or physically injured patients who are also contaminated. The contamination may be in the burn wound, and/or on or in the patient.

There are three common types of radiation: alpha, beta, and gamma rays. Alpha radiation is an internal hazard only; it cannot penetrate the intact skin and is not a hazard if kept out of the body. Beta radiation is the name given short-range, less-penetrating external radiation. Beta rays can be stopped by layers of clothing. Gamma radiation is the name given long-range, highly penetrating radiation. It consists of very short waves of pure energy traveling at the speed of light, is similar to x-rays, and can penetrate all but the densest materials. Two inches of lead, or thicker amounts of concrete, steel, water, or earth are shields for Gamma rays. Liquid or dust containing radiation can be a problem at the scene or in the hospital, causing a potential for contamination of the victim or immediate surroundings. Movement of people in the immediate area should be restricted until monitoring equipment is available.

There are, in general, three types of radiation hazards; external, internal, and contamination. By external radiation hazard is meant the exposure to a source of radiation which exists outside of the body. The x-ray machine is a familiar example of a source of external radiation. By internal radiation hazard is meant the exposure to radiation from radioactive materials which enter the body. Contamination is the presence of radioactive material where it is not desired.

A specific event or incident may involve all three categories of hazards. For example, a bottle of radioactive material would constitute an external hazard only. If, however, the material was spilled the area effected would be considered contaminated. If the radioactive material became airborne, then anyone entering the area would be breathing this material with a resulting internal hazard.

There are only three techniques for reducing the exposure from external sources. These techniques are: distance, time and shielding. When the distance between a relatively physically small source of radiation and the worker is increased, the worker takes advantage of the inverse square law. Thus, by doubling the distance from the source, the radiation intensity goes down and is reduced by a factor of four. If or when it is necessary to work in fields of more intense radiation, the exposure to the individual can be reduced by length of time spent in the radiation field. The third method of reducing external exposure is by the use of shielding between the source and the individual. Shielding is usually restricted to areas designed for radioactive material. For rescue and/or fire work advantage should be taken of any building structures as much as possible.

Radiation material can enter the body by ingestion, inhalation, absorption through cuts and breaks in the skin or direct absorption through the skin. The biological mechanism then takes over and its action depends upon the method of entry and the chemical and physical form of the radioactive material. Protective techniques include adequate ventilation, adequate respiratory protection and careful monitoring of clothing and body.

Any site where radiation materials are being stored or transferred will bear the familiar RADIATION WARNING SIGNAL. Chances are virtually nil that an accident involving dangerous radiation exposure should occur. However, hypothetical situations where there may be exposure to harmful radiation would be at a remote-site military crash or vehicle accident where contaminated materials are spilled, or an accident at a facility using radiation materials. An expert should be available at the scene of any such accident to measure contamination, direct handling of contaminated materials, etc. If one is not available Police should be directed to call Radiation Control Service at a University or Military Site in the area or the nearest hospital with Nuclear Medicine facilities. Rescue, however, should *NOT* be delayed waiting for such direction.

Medical personnel should not be responsible for directing decontamination, etc. Their primary responsibility is treatment; to remove the victim, and provide first aid. Police should see that someone is brought to the site with monitoring equipment to survey the site, everyone on the site and direct decontamination if needed. The medical worker should be aware of the safety precautions of time, distance, and shielding for him/her self and the victim.

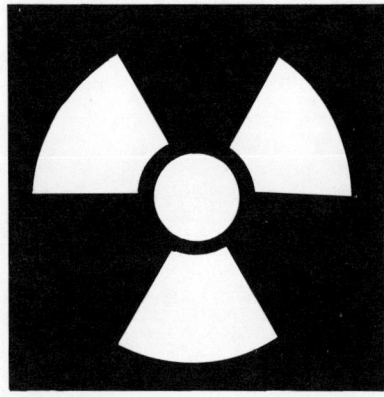

RADIATION WARNING SIGNAL

The primary responsibility of the rescue worker at the site of a radiation accident is to remove the victim from the contaminated field and provide first aid.

UNDER NO CIRCUMSTANCES SHOULD MEDICAL HELP BE WITHHELD BECAUSE OF POTENTIAL FOR RADIOACTIVE CONTAMINATION.

The priority of activities at the scene of the accident if radiation hazard is suspected and an expert is *not* available

to direct rescue are:[1]
- Instruct the police to contact a facility in the area with a Radiation Control Service to direct the scene.
- Call the nearest hospital with a Nuclear Medicine Department to alert a Nuclear Medicine physician that potentially radiation-contaminated victims will be taken to such and such an Emergency Department.
- Cover all body parts before entering exposure area with heavy clothing, gloves, shoes, etc.
- Wear a filtration mask if possible.
- Do not smoke or eat around radiation hazards (to prevent ingestion).
- **Get In and Get Out** is the rule. Stay as far away from the radiation source as possible. Use a shield if at all possible.
- Remove the victim as far from the radiation field as rapidly as possible.
- Provide first aid for respiratory or bleeding problems.
- Cover the patient and handle in a manner to limit possible spread of contamination from the patient and/or patients clothing.
- Transport immediately to an Emergency Department.
- Gather all details of the accident to assist in medical treatment.
- All rescuers and bystanders should stand by to be surveyed for radioactivity and decontaminated by the Radiation Control person once they arrive.
- **In Michigan, 24-hour information or assistance for radiation emergencies may be obtained by calling the nearest State Police Post or the Michigan State Police Operations Office in East Lansing, 1-517-373-0617.**

NOTE: Also consult Chapter 34, Radiation Exposure and Injury, Emergency Care and Transportation of the Sick and Injured, Committee on Injuries, American Academy of Orthopedic Surgeons, 1976.

Get in and get out is the rule of rescue of a radiation victim.

C. **First Aid for the Burned Victim: BREATHING, BLEEDING, SHOCK, Concurrent Injuries, and Severity of Burn**

Once the burning process has been stopped, *treat the burn victim as you would treat any trauma victim.* Forget the burn wound temporarily and begin systemic care. The burn wound itself is rarely life-threatening at the scene of the accident.

Treat the burn victim as you would any trauma victim.

---

[1] Possibilities for Improved Treatment of Persons Exposed in Radiation Accidents, Andrews, G.A.; Balish, E.; Edwards, C.L.; Kinseley, R.M.; Lushbaugh, C.C.; IAEA-SM-119/56.

EMERGENT CARE OF THE BURN VICTIM

However, the accident, explosion, fall or impact may result in life-threatening concurrent injuries. Though the burn wound is most obvious, treatment of other injuries takes priority. Definitive burn wound care is best delayed until the victim reaches the Emergency Department. Make a quick but thorough appraisal and treat *breathing, bleeding,* and *shock.* These important steps are begun at the scene of the accident and continue during transportation and after arrival in the Emergency Department.

Each step in first aid is dealt with individually in this text, even though they should be and usually are carried out simultaneously at the scene.

1. **Breathing: An Open AIRWAY is Essential to Survival**

    Objective: To ensure that the victim is obtaining oxygen in amounts adequate for brain, heart, lungs, and other organ systems to function.

    All organ systems require oxygen for function. A blocked airway stops oxygen supply. First aid always means FIRST—an open airway and adequate oxygen intake.

    The size of the burn wound does not necessarily determine the possibility of upper-airway or lower-lung involvement. In fact, some victims may have respiratory tract damage and have no obvious surface burns. Also, keep in mind that burn injury *does not* cause unconsciousness. *Find another cause!* Electrical and lightning injuries frequently cause cardio-pulmonary arrest. Those forced to breathe smoke while trapped in a burning room, car, etc., will have breathing problems. *Always suspect respiratory damage until all indicators are ruled out.*

    Upper airway problems are caused by trauma to and swelling of the mucous membrane lining in the nose and throat from absorption of heat and gases. Swelling in the upper airway causes obstruction and lack of oxygen intake. Lower airway or lung problems are due to prolonged exposure to heat and smoke. Lung damage interferes with oxygen exchange. Adequate oxygen intake is essential for both problems. Smoke inhalation victims also require oxygen and transport to the Emergency Department for evaluation and treatment. It is better to *administer oxygen when in doubt* than not to do so! Breathing difficulty may not be apparent until 24 hours later but oxygen at the scene does reduce the severity of the injury.

Always suspect respiratory damage until all indicators have been ruled out.

Adequate oxygen intake is essential. Administer oxygen when in doubt.

a. **Diagnosis**

Breathing difficulties include an evaluation of the following. *The presence of any of these indicates imminent respiratory problems:*
- Burned or trapped in an enclosed space; forced to breathe products of combustion. (House fire, car fire, or explosion.)
- Burns of the face and neck.
- Soot (carbon particles) on the mucosa of the nose and mouth.
- Singed nasal hairs.
- Obvious respiratory difficulty.
- Unconscious, disoriented, or decreased response or no response to stimuli.

ANY SUSPECTED OR APPARENT BREATHING DIFFICULTY REQUIRES IMMEDIATE TREATMENT.

b. **Treatment**

- Continue to talk to the victim to determine level of consciousness. (Obtain history of the accident from victim or bystanders.)
- Provide an open airway; remove false teeth; clear the mouth of foreign matter.
- Begin CPR if indicated. (Closed chest massage and mouth-to-mouth breathing, following accepted practice.)
- Administer precise concentrations of oxygen by tight-fitting face mask. (High concentrations of oxygen are essential if the patient is unconscious or has smoke inhalation damage.)
- Insert a tracheal or esophageal airway, if indicated, and *if trained* to do so.
- Elevate the head and torso if SHOCK is not present.
- Count the number of respirations per minute.
- Continue breathing support measures, begun at the scene of the accident, during transport. If manual CPR must be continued enroute, at least 3 rescuers plus a driver must accompany the victim—one for mouth-to-mouth, one for chest massage, and one to steady and relieve the one giving chest massage.

Administer precise concentrations of oxygen by tight fitting face mask.

2. **Evaluate BLEEDING: Head to Toe Survey**

   Objective: To detect and treat life-threatening injuries.

   As soon as an open airway is assured, conduct a rapid but thorough total body examination. A systematic head-to-toe review should be done and clothing removed from injured areas. Pulse, blood pressure, respiration, skin color and temperature, state of consciousness, ability to move, and response to pain indicate the need for specific therapy. These *basic diagnostic* signs can be checked in a short time with minimal equipment. Hemorrhage (internal or external), fractures, lacerations, head and/or neck injury and shock should be identified and treated according to accepted practice.

   The burn wound does not bleed — concurrent injury may cause bleeding.

   a. **Diagnosis**

   - Begin a systematic head-to-toe survey, checking for fractures, lacerations, head, neck, or spinal cord injury.
   - Determine the level of consciousness, response to pain, ability to move.
   - Check pulse, blood pressure, respirations for signs of internal injury.
   - Check skin color and temperature.
   - Cut away clothes from injured areas.

   b. **Treatment**

   - Treat hemorrhage, lacerations, fractures, spinal cord injury, etc., according to accepted medical practice.

3. **Shock—CIRCULATORY System Failure**

   Objective: To ensure circulation adequate to carry oxygen to the brain, lungs, heart, and other organ systems.

   In any trauma victim, transport of oxygen to organ systems may be reduced through lack of circulating blood volume. This is called shock. Shock may be neurogenic due to action of the nervous system, cardiogenic due to decreased heart action, or hypovolemic due to loss of circulating blood volume. Initially, the shock experienced by the burn victim will be neurogenic—a normal body response to trauma or crisis. The patient may be anxious, cool and clammy from perspiration, or may exhibit no symptoms. However, if the victim is severely injured, life-threatening shock may be imminent.

The body's normal response to the burn injury is inflammation; fluid shifts out of the bloodstream into injured tissues. This fluid shift begins immediately post-injury, and if the burn is greater than 15 to 20% total body area, the gradual result is an insufficient amount of circulating blood. Unless there is associated hemorrhage, the fluid shift is not immediately life-threatening; however, if proper treatment does not take place within a few hours, the outcome will be hypovolemic shock and death. In the severely burned patient this is termed **burn shock**.

Treatment of hypovolemic shock best takes place in a hospital because large volumes of closely monitored IV fluids are needed. If the EMT is trained, an IV with Ringer's lactate solution may be started at the scene; however, little damage from burn shock will occur without an IV if transport is rapid. If there is severe bleeding from concurrent injuries or transport must be delayed, an IV should be started; BP, P, R closely monitored, and when possible, radio contact for instruction maintained with a physician.

Treatment of hypovolemic shock best takes place in a hospital.

Note: Keep in mind that if an IV is inserted, the flow rate should be slow to moderate at the scene and enroute, because more damage than good can be done to the victim's heart and lungs by overloading them with IV fluids.

a. **Diagnosis**

- Check blood pressure, pulse, respiration, skin color, and temperature.
- Symptoms of shock:
    - blood pressure below 100/ systolic.
    - pulse over 120 per minute.
    - respirations rapid and shallow — 16 to 28 per minute.
    - skin cool and clammy.

b. **Treatment**

- If shock is detected, have the patient lie flat.
- Cover the victim with a blanket.
- Begin IV therapy *only if:*
    - **the burn is greater than 20% total body area;**

Do not give oral fluids.

    → there are associated injuries and on instructions of a physician; and,
    → **trained to do so.**
  • Start 1,000 ml lactated Ringer's (Hartmann's), run in slowly. **A physician should direct flow rate.**
  • *Do not* give oral fluids unless the patient is alert, can swallow, has no internal injuries, and has *only very minor burns.* Oral fluids given to a patient with large burns may cause vomiting or aspiration.
  • Treatment for shock is best begun in the Emergency Department.
   Note: Because the fluid reserves in a child or the aged are limited, immediate transport is essential.

 D. **Severity of Burn**

  1. <u>Diagnosis</u>

Burn wound care at the scene is simply prevention of further trauma.

   All burns are not alike. Table III detailed the difference between a minor and major burn. Care at the scene of the accident is basically the same for both injuries, and both should be transported to the Emergency Department. Treatment which may be given at the scene for a very superficial injury with no other trauma is also detailed below.

   Infection control is important in care of the burn wound. However, first aid infection control measures require no more than *prevention of additional contamination.* Wet dressings only serve as a wick to pull bacteria into the wound. Peeling off or removing clothing that has melted into the wound only causes further damage. Delaying transport to the hospital while putting on sterile gown and gloves, and applying wet sterile dressings only delays further life-saving measures and provides very little benefit to the wound. Burn wound care at the scene is simply prevention of further trauma.

  2. **Major Burn Wound Treatment**

   Objective: To protect the burn wound from further trauma and infection.

  • Remove clothing over the burn wound if not adherent.
   → Make no attempt to remove adherent clothing,

especially melted material, such as synthetic clothing, from the wound unless this is absolutely necessary to stop the burning process or to treat concurrent injuries.
- Quickly estimate percent of burn using Rule of Nines (refer to Figure 2).
- Do not apply any ointments, solutions, or dressings to the burn wound unless they are to stop bleeding.
  - → No sterile gloves or gowns required.
  - → Clean technique is acceptable. Stringent infection control measures will begin in the hospital.
  - → Wet dressings are *not* indicated; they may act as a wick, pulling bacteria into the wound.
- Wrap the victim in a clean, dry, or sterile sheet.
- Cover the victim with a blanket.
  - → Avoid drafts, prevent cooling, keep warm.
- Transfer to a stretcher for transport.

Wrap the victim in a clean, dry or sterile sheet.

3. **Superficial Minor Burns (Treatment at the Scene of the Accident)**

   Objective: To prepare the minor wound for spontaneous healing.

   Care of a minor burn involves all of the above considerations and may also require transport to an Emergency Department. However, if all of the above first aid measures have been considered and ruled out, and a very small superficial burn is the only injury (less than 1% of the body), care is as follows:

   A superficial minor burn covers less than 1% of the body with NO other severity factors.

   - Gently cleanse the wound and adjacent area of all soot, dirt, and debris with soap and tap water.
   - Shave any hair in and around the wound.
   - Rinse thoroughly with tap water.
   - Cover the wound with a sterile bandage.
   - Instruct the victim to see his/her family physician or Emergency Department physician as soon as possible (within 24 hours) for evaluation of tetanus coverage and further wound care.

E. **Mass Casualties**

   Objective: To provide immediate lifesaving treatment to as many victims as possible.

   When confronted with a disaster resulting in a number of

burn victims, keep in mind the principle of *systemic treatment first:* FIRST AID for the severely injured. Treatment of the burn wound is not begun until all lifesaving measures have been taken. *The size of the burn wound, and part of the body burned, however, are a consideration in therapy.* Burns of the face, neck and chest may indicate immediate or impending respiratory difficulty. An extensive wound, over 20% of the body, indicates imminent shock and need for fluids.

Provide an open airway and administer oxygen.

- Make a rapid appraisal for those requiring immediate respiratory assistance.
- Provide an open airway and oxygen.
- Determine life-threatening lacerations, fractures, and obvious or internal hemorrhage, and size of burn, using Rule of Nines.
- Provide appropriate first aid.
- Begin an IV to delay shock, if indicated, if transport to an Emergency Department cannot be done immediately, and *if* the EMT is trained. (See Diagnosis and Treatment of Shock.)
- Transport the victims (priority given to the most severely injured) to the Emergency Department as soon as possible.

F. Emotional Support

Objective: To assist the victim to cope with this crisis situation.

In addition to and while providing life support measures, keep in mind that the burn victim is an accident victim. Pain and fear of disfigurement and dying may be overwhelming. Guilt regarding the cause of the accident and anxiety for loved ones may add to the fear. The patient requires reassurance and support to cope with this crisis situation. Your calm and effective first aid measures provide a feeling of confidence, but also important is your assurance that you are administering the best possible care.

Talk to the victim, explain what you are doing and what you want him/her to do.

- Speak calmly to the victim.
- Acknowledge the victim's primary complaint.
- *Explain briefly what you are doing and why, and what you expect the victim to do.*
- Assure the victim that he/she is receiving the best first aid and will be transported to further care as soon as possible.
- Talk *to* the victim, not *about* him/her.
- Answer questions regarding the accident, friends, and family

in a reassuring manner.
- Do not discuss the ultimate severity of the victim's injuries or those of others with the victim.
- Explain to family and/or friends what is being done, where the victim is to be transferred, and what they may do.

G. <u>Transportation to an Emergency Department</u>

Objective: Immediate transport of the victim to intensive medical care while continuing the life-saving measures begun at the scene of the accident.

Traditionally, transport of an accident victim to the Emergency Department has been the primary role of the emergency worker. This role has been expanded to provide excellence in care at the scene of the accident, which will reduce the severity of the injury and ensure that the patient arrives at the Emergency Department with lifesaving measures already underway. Transportation to definitive care remains a primary goal of the EMT. Once you have assured that the victim is breathing adequately, not bleeding, and has been treated to delay or avoid shock, transport the victim to the nearest hospital providing emergency care. If the burn or frostbite victim has concurrent injuries, such as head injury, fractures, or spinal injuries, transportation requires immobilization in accordance with accepted first aid practice to prevent further and possibly more severe injury.

- Follow established EMS communications patterns with the Emergency Department.
- Continue enroute all first aid measures begun at the scene of the accident!
- Check vital signs: blood pressure, pulse, and respiration at least once.
- If the patient has respiratory involvement, place on side with the head elevated (rather than prone) during transportation, to assist in maintaining an open airway. (Elevate head only if blood pressure is 100/systolic or above.)
- Provide emotional support and reassurance.
- Organize the events of the accident and first aid given at the scene.
- Complete any necessary forms.

Continue enroute all life saving measures begun at the scene of the accident.

H. <u>Transition to Care in the Emergency Department</u>

The EMT's responsibility are not relieved when the victim

The EMT's responsibilities are not relieved until care in the Emergency Department is begun.

reaches the Emergency Department. Continuity of care begun at the scene of the accident and a smooth transition to Emergency Department care are essential.

Care in the Emergency Department consists of a repeat appraisal of the injury and indepth first aid. Intubation or tracheostomy may be necessary to maintain an open airway and provide oxygen, and definitive treatment is begun for concurrent injuries and shock. The severity of the injury is systematically determined, based on the extent of burn, concurrent injuries, age, and medical history. The appropriate level of burn care is determined by these severity factors. Wound care may again be delayed until after transfer to a specialized burn care facility.

A concise, accurate account of the injury, victim's condition, and care at the scene of the accident are essential to providing excellence in care in the Emergency Department.

- Continue life support measures in the Emergency Department until instructed to stop.
- Give the attending physician (or nurse) a brief but thorough description of the accident, treatment given at the scene of the accident, and enroute, and any specific observations pertinent to treatment. (Review III, A, 1 in next section.)
- Determine (from physician) the need for transport of the victim (within a short period) to a specialized burn care facility.

III. CARE OF THE BURN VICTIM IN THE EMERGENCY DEPARTMENT

Care from the time of the accident to successful resuscitation is termed emergent period care. Care in the emergent period is life-saving, as well as preparatory for definitive therapy. Attention to detail can make the difference between life and death. The initial treatment given the severely burned patient at the scene of the accident and in the Emergency Department serves as the foundation on which continuing excellence in care is built. The principles of care for this period, in order of importance are:

Care in the Emergency Department is not only life saving but also lays the foundation for excellence in continued care.

- First Aid.
- Fluid Therapy.
- Wound Care.
- Considerations for Safety and Further Therapy.

First aid is a continuous process throughout the emergent period of care: begun at the scene of the accident, continued and expanded in the Emergency Department, and completed at the specialized burn care facility. Once the patient has been stabilized the emergent period of care ends.

The *EMS Burn Care Poster* shown in Figure 4 serves as a basis for this section of Emergency Department care. It has been prepared by the National Institute for Burn Medicine as a part of the Burn Information and Triage System (BITS). This poster, manual, training film, and the Information Phone System, 313-995-BURN, provide a total system for excellence in burn care from the scene of the accident to specialized care.

A. First Aid in the Emergency Department (Box 1, EMS Poster)

Arrival of the burn victim in the Emergency Department presents problems similar to other types of trauma and is the signal for a second assessment of the need for first aid. *The burn victim is a trauma victim; both require the same first aid measures.* The burn is obvious; however, a quick but careful

Arrival by the victim in the Emergency Department signals the need for FIRST AID.

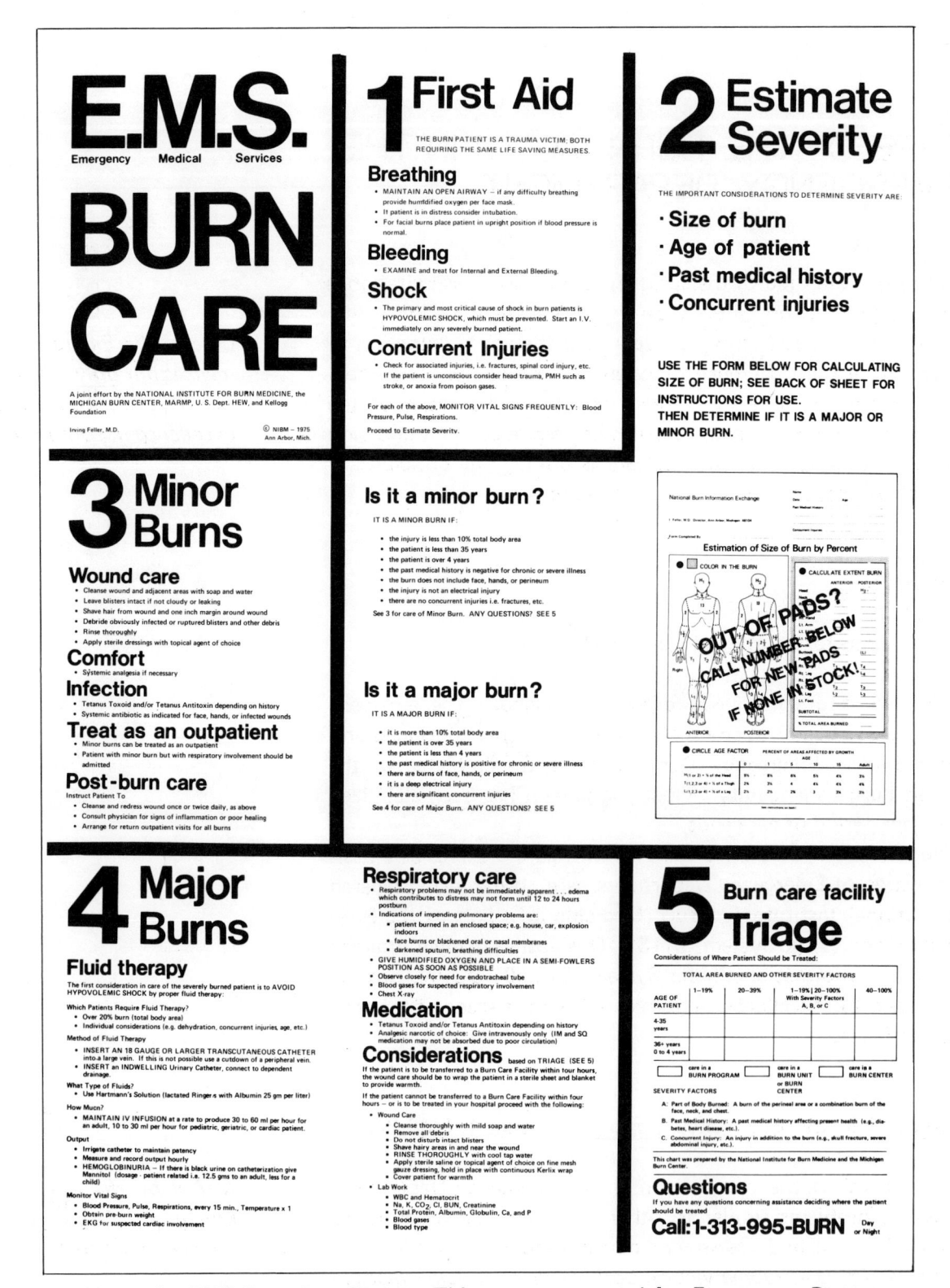

Figure 4. EMS Burn Care Poster. This poster, prepared for Emergency Department use, serves as an outline of care to be discussed in the section on Emergency Department care of the burned victim.

search for other (concurrent) injuries must be made and appropriate therapy initiated. When administering first aid to any seriously injured patient, *breathing, bleeding,* and *shock* are paramount considerations, usually in that order. Vital signs, blood pressure, pulse, respiratory rate, and temperature should be carefully taken and recorded frequently.

Assess the victim for:
- *Breathing*
- *Bleeding*
- *Shock*

Although many of the following procedures occur simultaneously when a medical team works on a patient, each is discussed individually to provide proper emphasis.

1. Transition of Care

    It is important for the Emergency Department staff to obtain, before the EMT leaves, an accurate history of the accident and emergency treatment already given. To provide a smooth transition of care:

    - Instruct the EMT to continue or stop therapy.
    - Obtain the following information from the EMT:
        - Name and address of patient.
        - A description and cause of the accident.
        - Rescue measures preceding emergency care.
        - Condition of the patient at the scene.
        - Details of emergency care at the scene and during transport.
        - Any relevant observation of response to trauma or treatment.
        - For legal purposes, make special note of neglect, homicide, inflicted injury, or suicide details.
        - Disposition of patient's valuables.
    - Instruct the EMT as to need for further transportation, i.e., to a specialized burn care facility.

2. Stop the Burning Process

    Even though the burning process should have been eliminated at the scene of the accident, it is important to repeat this step. (Review pages 12 thru 19.)

    Make a brief but careful search for smoldering clothing, chemicals, or other burning agents.

    - Make a brief but careful search for smoldering clothing, chemicals, or other burning agents.

    a. Thermal

        - Remove all clothing. If clothing is adherent to the wound:
            - Soak with saline (mixed 1:1 with peroxide if

necessary) then remove.
- If clothing is drenched with gasoline, or other flammable liquid, remove and wrap in plastic bag to prevent further ignition.

b. **Chemical**

FLUSH CHEMICAL INJURY WITH COPIOUS AMOUNTS OF WATER.

- Flush chemical injuries with copious amounts of water.
- Determine the type of chemical.
- See Table IV for details of neutralization of a chemical injury. (Many authorities feel neutralization only serves to produce increased trauma and recommend copious water lavage.)
- If there is a question on how to treat a specific chemical injury, call the Burn Information number or your local Poison Control Center.
- Also review page 14 in the previous section for details on handling chemical injury.
- Call an Ophthalmologist if eyes are involved.

c. **Tar Burns**

Hot tar coats the injured area and cannot be adequately removed unless the tar has been hardened. Immersion of the tar-coated area in ice water hardens the tar and it may then be peeled from the injured area.

- Immerse the body area in ice water for a few minutes (not longer than 3).
- Remove the area from the ice water and peel the hardened tar from the wound.
- It is not essential that *all* tar be removed from the wound in the Emergency Department. Tar embedded in the wound can be removed at the burn care facility by repeat dressing changes. (Some authorities recommend *lard* or petrolatum applied to the tar for removal. If ice water does not suffice, this method may be tried.)

d. **Electrical**

Search for electrical entry and exit wounds; e.g., groin, antecubital, and popliteal spaces.

There will be an entry and exit wound which may be very small but deep. There also may be a thermal burn if clothing ignited. (See page 14.)

e. **Frostbite** (See page 62)

National Institute for Burn Medicine — EMERGENT CARE OF THE BURN VICTIM

TABLE IV

EMERGENT TREATMENT OF CHEMICAL BURNS

AGENT and TREATMENT	TISSUE TOXICITY
Oxidizing agents	
1. Chromic acid → a. Dilute → b. Wash w/dilute Na hyposulfite → c. British anti lewisite dimercaprol (BAL) for systemic toxicity	5-10g lethal; coagulates protein, ulcerates and blisters w/perforation nasal septum; ulcerates skin and coagulates
2. Chlorox (Na-hypochlorite) → a. Milk, eggwhite, starch paste → b. Lavage → c. Na thiosulfate 1% solution	Releases free chlorine, coagulates protein
3. Potassium permanganate → a. Liberal lavage → b. Eggwhite	Potent oxidizer producing thick, brownish purple eschar of coagulated protein
Reducing agents	
1. Alkyl mercury agents → a. Debride → b. Remove blister fluid → c. Lavage	5-50 mg/kg lethal; redness, bleb formation, partial-thickness lesions which deepen if blister fluid is not evacuated
2. HCL (see also E2 below) → a. Avoid lavage → b. Neutralize with soda lime, soap-magnesium hydroxide → c. Demulcents	Rapid conversion of protein to coagulum salt of the acid; shallow ulcers form with coagulated eschar and base, prolonged action depending on exposure concentration
3. HNO_3	
Corrosives	
1. Phenol (cresol) → a. Dilute w/water or cover w/oil; avoid alcohol → b. Demulcents → c. May use activated charcoal p.o.	Soft, white coagulum caused by protein denaturization, absorption rapid
2. Phosphorous (white) → a. Lavage with: $KMnO_4$ 1:5000 or → b. $Cu(SO_4)$ 2% or → c. Cover w/oil	50-100 mg lethal, soluble in oils, fumes and for burns as becomes P_2O_3
3. Dichromate salts → a. Lavage w/water → b. 2% hyposulfite wash → c. Lavage w/buffer of 7% (w/w) KH_2PO_4: 18% (w/w) Na_2HPO_4 : H_2O (70 g : 180 g : 850 ml4)	10g lethal, highly corrosive to skin and mucosa; soft yellow coagulum and indolent, deep ulceration; long action
4. Sodium metal; lye • Lyes KOH NaOH NH_4OH LiOH $Ba_2(OH)_3$ $Ca(OH)_3$ → a. Dilute with lavage → b. Neutralize with weak acid → c. Demulcents → d. Appropriate systemic therapy	(Also see Salt Formers) Liquefaction necrosis, soft, gelatinous, brown, friable tissue destruction; fulminant initial response; supporting structures often left intact; saponify fats, salt out collagen, dehydrate other cells
• Na_2 → a. Cover with oil → b. Avoid water → c. Excise	In presence of water forms NaOH and heat, and may explode
D. **Protoplasmic poisons**	
1. Salt formers Tungstic acid Picric acid Sulfosalicylic acid Tannic acid Trichloroacetic acid Cresylic acid Acetic acid Formic acid → a. Liberal water lavage → b. Demulcents → c. Cover w/oil	5-50 mg/kg lethal; form the homologous proteinate when in contact with tissue; escharotic; firm to hard eschar with some sparing of underlying support structures occurs; may be absorbed and produce hepatotoxicity and/or nephrotoxicity; acetic is especially penetrating, formic especially long-lived.
2. Metabolic competitor/inhibitor Oxalic acid → a. Immediate admin. soluble Ca^{++} salt solution in large volume → b. Careful lavage → c. I.V. calcium → d. ? parathormone I.V.	15-30g lethal; affects mucous membrane; chalk white indolent ulcer; acts by binding Ca^{++} and poisoning protoplasm
3. Hydrofluoric acid → a. Boric acid wash → b. $NaHCO_3$ wash → c. Local infiltration of Ca gluconate → d. Local $MgSO_4$ paste and/or Hyamine 0.2% in iced alcohol or water	± 1.5g lethal, painful, indolent; deep ulcerations below tough coagulum
E. **Desiccants**	
1. H_2SO_4 → a. Avoid water lavage → b. Neutralize with magnesium oxide, lime water, soap → c. Demulcents	Potent desiccant, produces hard eschar with indolent ulcer, deep destruction of all carbon-containing tissue; liberates considerable heat during reaction
2. Muriatic acid (conc. HCl-commercial grade) → a. See H_2SO_4 and B2 above	Slower coagulation process than H_2SO_4, but produces deeper, more severe ulcers and less heat; otherwise lesions similar
F. **Vesicants**	
1. Cantharides → a. Water lavage → b. Avoid oils	5-50 mg/kg lethal; potent vesicant; severe partial-thickness lesions (Spanish Fly)
2. DMSO → a. Water lavage	22g lethal; causes hemolysis, histamine and serotonin release, edema, ischemia, water soluble
3. Mustard gas → a. Wash w/oil, kerosene or gasoline, then soap and water	Severe blistering and partial-thickness necrosis of skin and mucosa; vesicles form, breakdown @ 24-48 hr, then ulcerate
4. Lewisite → a. BAL	0.1 mg/kg lethal, same actions as mustard gas, but slower action

After: Table I., Chemicals That "Burn"; <u>Chemicals That Burn</u>, Jelenko, Carl III; Journal of Trauma 14:1, January 1974.

f. **Radiation**

Radiation injuries may be grouped in two types. The first are those injuries from X-ray, Gamma rays or ionizing radiation. Once the victim is removed from the radiation source there is no immediate problem, the victim or rescuer is not rendered radioactive. The victims of such exposure can develop life threatening complications later. Although their problems are not immediate, these victims may require treatment for hematopoietic, gastrointestinal, central nervous system and skin problems. These complications may be fatal and it is this type of accident where reenactment of the scene may be necessary to determine the internal dosage. The only care required in the Emergency Department for such accidents other than usual first aid measures, is an accurate history of the accident and an immediate complete blood count (especially a WBC to monitor leukocyte change) to serve as a baseline for future care.

The second group of victims are those not only exposed to radiation but who have also had a radioactive substance deposited on their clothing or person, which may continue to contaminate the environment in which they are handled and is a continuing source of radiation exposure to the victim and possibly others. These patients require someone *on site* in the Emergency Department with a working knowledge of handling radioactivity. In the ED the victim, his clothes, objects, and movement of those caring for him should be restricted, i.e., to one room or small area. The victim however, should have any medical problem treated *as if there were no* radiation involvement. Radiation badges should be worn by care personnel, if available, but treatment should *NOT* be delayed waiting for badges. Clothing, excrement, vomitus, hair, feces, urine, blood, etc., should be contained and labeled until it can be surveyed. If a wound should be contaminated, surgical debridement is indicated to remove the contaminated material, eg., radioactive metallic powder. Emergency medical personnel and vehicles which transported the victim should be retained until they can be surveyed for possible radioactivity. Clothing, blankets, sheets, scrub clothes, etc., which may be potentially radioactive should also be plastic bagged, labeled, and

The radiation accident victim should have any medical problem treated as if there were NO radioactivity.

retained until they can be surveyed.

Medical personnel should not be responsible for guessing about contamination and decontamination. A physician from the Nuclear Medicine Department of the hospital or an "expert" from Radiation Control Service from a nearby military site or University should be brought in with monitoring equipment to survey the victim and scene, and direct care and decontamination.

Medical personnel should not be responsible for guessing about radioactive contamination and decontamination.

In the instance of potentially radioactive victims:

- Review page 16 on Radiation Injuries (Care at the Scene).
- <u>Call for a physician from the nearest hospital Nuclear Medicine Department for consultation.</u>
- Call for and wear radiation badges.
- Assign the victim(s) to one area for care (contain all activity of victim and care personnel to that area) until survey and decontamination can be done.
- Assign one/two persons to care *only* for that victim.
- Handle contaminated patient and wound as you would a surgical procedure; i.e., gown, gloves, cap, mask, etc.
- **Provide first aid (life support and wound care measures) as required.**
- Instruct EMT's and vehicle and/or stretcher to stand by until monitoring (and decontamination) can be completed.
- Obtain an accurate history of the accident.
- Obtain blood sample for WBC/CBC.
- Retain all clothing, metal objects (eg. jewelery), vomitus, hair, feces, blood, urine, blankets, etc., for monitoring. (Double bag and label with patients name, date and RADIOACTIVE – DO NOT DISCARD.)
- Save all nurses, physicians, and attendents scrub clothing etc., after use, double bag and label as above.
- Follow instructions of Radiation Control person as to decontamination.

A handbook which the Emergency Department staff may find useful is <u>Emergency Handling of Radiation Cases</u>, U.S. Atomic Energy Commission, 1969.

EMERGENT CARE OF THE BURN VICTIM — National Institute for Burn Medicine

3. **First Aid**

The burn wound, though most obvious, is not immediately life-threatening. Concurrent injuries may be. *Care of the burn wound follows first aid.*

Care of the burn wound follows first aid.

- Remove dressings and clothing; cover patient with clean sheet for warmth and modesty.
- Make a brief but thorough head to toe search for injuries.
- Determine level of consciousness. **The burn injury does not render the victim unconscious.** Search for other causes.
- Administer accepted first aid for breathing, bleeding, shock, and concurrent injuries.

a. **Airway (Immediate Respiratory Care)**

The first step in care of any trauma victim is to establish an open airway and adequate oxygen intake.

Provide an open airway and adequate oxygen intake.

- Remove debris and open the airway.
- Suction the nasopharynx and trachea as indicated.
- Determine need for and entubate and/or initiate cardio-pulmonary resuscitation (CPR), if the airway is obstructed.
- Provide precise concentrations of humidified oxygen.
- Obtain baseline blood gases for any suspicion of pulmonary problems.
- Elevate the head of the bed if the victim is not hypotensive.
- Stay with the patient.
- See Care of Major Burn (Box 4, EMS Poster) for details of care for respiratory involvement.

b. **Bleeding**

Treat concurrent injury.

The burn injury itself does not result in either internal or external bleeding. Concurrent injury from the accident, such as laceration, fracture, etc., may cause external bleeding. A fall, impact, or explosion may cause internal injuries such as spleen or liver rupture. First aid treatment of these injuries is not different for a burn victim than another trauma victim.

- Make a brief, thorough check for external bleeding.
- Control external bleeding through accepted practices.
- Examine the chest and abdomen for possible internal injuries.
- Check blood pressure, pulse, and respiratory rate every 15 minutes as indicators of internal injuries.
- Obtain x-rays as indicated.
- Check the hematocrit as an indicator of internal injuries.
- Perform peritoneal lavage for question of abdominal bleeding based on x-ray and physical diagnosis.

c. **Shock**

The primary and most critical cause of shock in the severely burned victim is hypovolemia, which results in hypovolemic shock and death if not treated with proper fluid replacement.

- Start an IV immediately through a large bore catheter into a deep vein, or any available vein.
- See Care of Major Burns for further discussion of fluid therapy.

Start an IV through a large bore catheter immediately.

d. **Concurrent Injuries**

If the burn injury involved a fall, impact, or explosion, concurrent injuries must be considered.

- Make a brief, careful head-to-toe examination for possible concurrent injuries.
- Check for fractures, spinal cord injury, etc.
- Consider head trauma, stroke, or anoxia from poisonous gases if the patient is unconscious.
- Administer oxygen in precise concentrations to the unconscious patient.
- Follow accepted emergency procedures for care of concurrent injuries.

A burn injury does not render the patient unconscious. FIND another cause.

4. **Emotional Support**

It is important to keep in mind that the burn victim is an accident victim. The patient will have guilt feelings regarding the accident, possibly have a fear of death, or, at least, a fear of the "unknown" concerning the injury and treatment. The shock and the pain of the accident, the chaos and rush to the hospital, the unknown surroundings and the people, all add up to emotional stress.

An attitude of confidence, genuine interest, and concern are extremely important to the emotional welfare of the patient and family. **One simple act which provides an anchor in the storm is for the nurse or physician to tell the patient his/her name and to explain briefly what to expect of the staff and what will be expected of the patient.** These instructions (a contract) eliminate the inequality and inconsistency in the transition from citizen to victim to patient. Talking to the patient also allows the medical worker to evaluate the patient's sensorium and orientation.

Tell the patient your name, call him/her by name. Explain what will be done and what you want the patient to do.

- Give the patient your name and call the patient by name.
- **Talk to the patient**, not just "about him".
- State what will be done and why.
- Request the patient's cooperation and suggest possible ways of participation.
- Encourage the patient to express his/her feelings and alter the contract to comply with the patient's requests when possible.
- Take time when life-saving activities are complete to notify a relative or friend of the victim, and discuss the patient's disposition and give them instructions on what must be done.
- Assure the victim that his relatives (or friends) have been kept abreast of his condition.

B. <u>Estimation of Severity of the Injury (Box 2, EMS Poster)</u>

All burns are not alike. Treatment is related to severity.

All burns are not alike. A first considerations in care is an accurate determination of severity of injury. Treatment is directly related to severity. Severity factors are also considered when determining the level of continued care required by the victim. Influencing severity of injury are five factors: (1) extent of burn, (2) depth of injury, (3) age, (4) past medical history, (5) part of body injured, including concurrent injuries.

1. <u>Extent of Burn</u>

Extent of burn is expressed as a percentage of total body area. A fairly standardized and accurate method of determining extent of burn is illustrated in Figure 5 and is the same as described in the EMS Burn Care Poster, Box 2.

It is important to refer to the diagram and burn wound and accurately map out the injury. <u>Underestimation may result in lack of treatment. Overestimation results in overzealous therapy, especially in the child</u>, geriatric, cardiac, or victim with respiratory injury. Keep in mind while estimating difficult areas that the entire palm of the victim's hand represents 1% of the body.

Accurately estimate the percent of body burned.

- Using the diagram on the EMS poster (Box 2), determine the percentage of body burned (burn size).

2. **Depth of Burn**

Depth of burn is difficult to determine and is not extremely important to emergency care, but does affect survival and is considered in specialized care. Signs and symptoms help indicate the level of tissue damage, but only with demarcation and spontaneous healing or appearance of granulation tissue can the exact depth of injury and destruction be determined. Depth of burn is best described in terms of partial-thickness or full-thickness. These are anatomically descriptive and preferable to popular references to first and second degree (partial-thickness) and third degree (full-thickness) burns—terms which arose from visual impressions. In a partial-thickness burn the tissue damage and destruction do not include the deeper dermal layers, and with good care new skin is regenerated. In a full-thickness burn, the skin and its appendages have been destroyed and the subcutaneous tissue, muscle, and bone may be damaged. Skin grafting is necessary to replace the destroyed tissues. Figure 6 describes the factors of differential diagnosis of depth of burn.

Depth of burn is difficult to accurately determine immediately post burn.

In general, the patient who has a painful, erythematous surface with vesicles probably has a partial-thickness burn. Where there is no complaint of pain and the surface is anesthetic, a full-thickness burn usually exists.

3. **Age**

Age is an important factor in determining severity of injury. Figure 7 demonstrates that patients less than 4 and more than 35 years of age have a higher mortality rate than other age groups with similar size injury. Essentially, the problem in the infant and youngster is poor

Age of the patient can affect survival.

EMERGENT CARE OF THE BURN VICTIM — National Institute for Burn Medicine

FIGURE 5

ESTIMATION OF SIZE OF BURN BY PERCENT

INSTRUCTIONS FOR COMPLETING FORM

❶ COLOR IN THE BURN
Shade or color in the body diagrams to represent as closely as possible how the burn looks to you when viewing the patient from directly anterior and/or directly posterior. Ignore the dashed lines on the diagrams while doing this.

❷ CIRCLE AGE FACTOR
Since body proportions change from infancy to adulthood and since these changes mainly affect relative head and lower extremity proportions, this table allows you to choose the most appropriate body proportions for the age of the patient. Ages 0, 1, 5, 10, 15 and adult are given. Choose the age closest to that of the patient and use the H (head), T (thigh) and L (leg) percentage factors in the column below the age selected. To avoid mistakes, circle these numbers.

❸ CALCULATE EXTENT BURN
Each body part listed in the calculation table is indicated on the anterior and posterior body diagrams by dashed lines. The percentage of total body surface area for each body part is printed either on the diagram or in the age factor table (step 2). If the shaded or colored area in the body diagram covers an entire body part, the whole percentage figure for that part is entered into the calculation table. If the shaded area covers only a fraction of a body part, then that fraction of the percentage figure is entered. For example, if an anterior chest burn covered about one-third of the trunk, then 1/3 of 13, or 4% would be entered in the space for "trunk (anterior)". When all body parts have been considered, subtotals are made for anterior and posterior of total body area burned. This number is most frequently referred to as the "size of the burn".

NATIONAL BURN INFORMATION EXCHANGE

I. Feller, M.D. Director, Ann Arbor, Michigan 48104

Name: _____
Date: _____ Age: _____
Past Medical History: _____
Form Completed By: _____
Concurrent Injuries: _____

Estimation of Size of Burn by Percent

❶ COLOR IN THE BURN

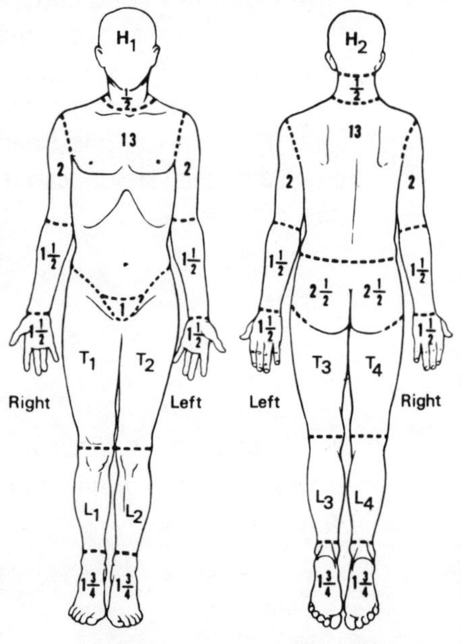

❸ CALCULATE EXTENT BURN

	ANTERIOR	POSTERIOR
Head	H₁	H₂
Neck		
Rt. Arm		
Rt. Forearm		
Rt. Hand		
Lt. Arm		
Lt. Forearm		
Lt. Hand		
Trunk		
Buttock	(R)	(L)
Perineum		
Rt. Thigh	T₁	T₄
Rt. Leg	L₁	L₄
Rt. Foot		
Lt. Thigh	T₂	T₃
Lt. Leg	L₂	L₃
Lt. Foot		
SUBTOTAL		
% TOTAL AREA BURNED		%

❷ CIRCLE AGE FACTOR PERCENT OF AREAS AFFECTED BY GROWTH

AGE	0	1	5	10	15	Adult
H (1 or 2) = ½ of the Head	9½	8½	6½	5½	4½	3½
T (1,2,3 or 4) = ½ of a Thigh	2¾	3¼	4	4¼	4½	4¾
L (1,2,3 or 4) = ½ of a Leg	2½	2½	2¾	3	3¼	3½

(see instructions on back)

40

DIFFERENTIAL DIAGNOSIS OF DEPTH OF BURN

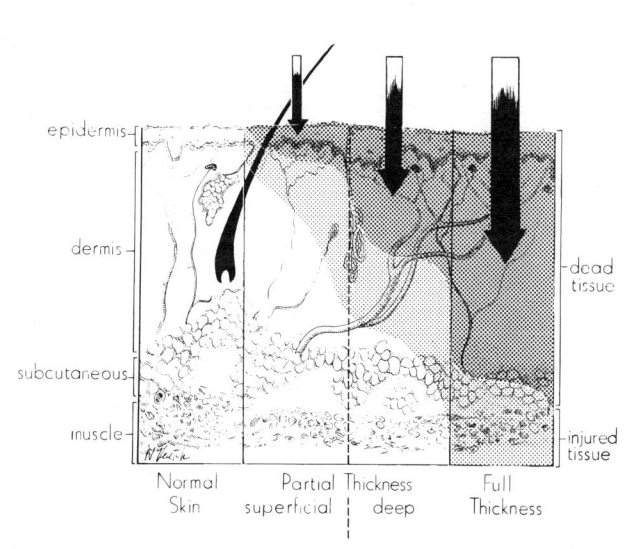

Figure 6. Depth of Burn. The arrows represent degree of *heat* or intensity of burning agent, and the *time* of contact with skin. The darker shaded area represents dead tissue; the lighter shaded area, damaged or injured tissue which will heal with good care. When all tissue (epidermis and dermis) has been destroyed, this is termed full-thickness. Partial-thickness means only part of the skin has been destroyed. Damaged tissue can reheal with good care.

DIFFERENTIAL DIAGNOSIS

PARTIAL—THICKNESS BURN		FULL—THICKNESS BURN
Normal or increased sensitivity to pain and temperature	Sensation	Anesthetic to pain and temperature
Large, thick-walled, will usually increase in size	Blisters	None, or if present, thin-walled and will not increase in size
Red, will blanch with pressure and refill	Color	White, brown, black or red. If red, will not blanch with pressure
Normal or firm	Texture	Firm or leathery

EMERGENT CARE OF THE BURN VICTIM National Institute for Burn Medicine

FIGURE 7

National Burn Information Exchange
BURNED PATIENT SURVIVAL BY AGE GROUP
Percent Total Area Burned

I. Feller, Director, Ann Arbor, Michigan

Survival Curves Fit By Probit Analysis For Age Groups:
- 5-34 Years - 5520 cases
- 2-4, 35-49 Years - 3254
- 0-1, 50-59 Years - 2275
- 60-74 Years - 601
- 75-100 Years - 233

Total Number of Cases - 11,883 - from 1966-1973 statistics (NBIE)

PERCENT SURVIVAL

PERCENT TOTAL AREA BURNED

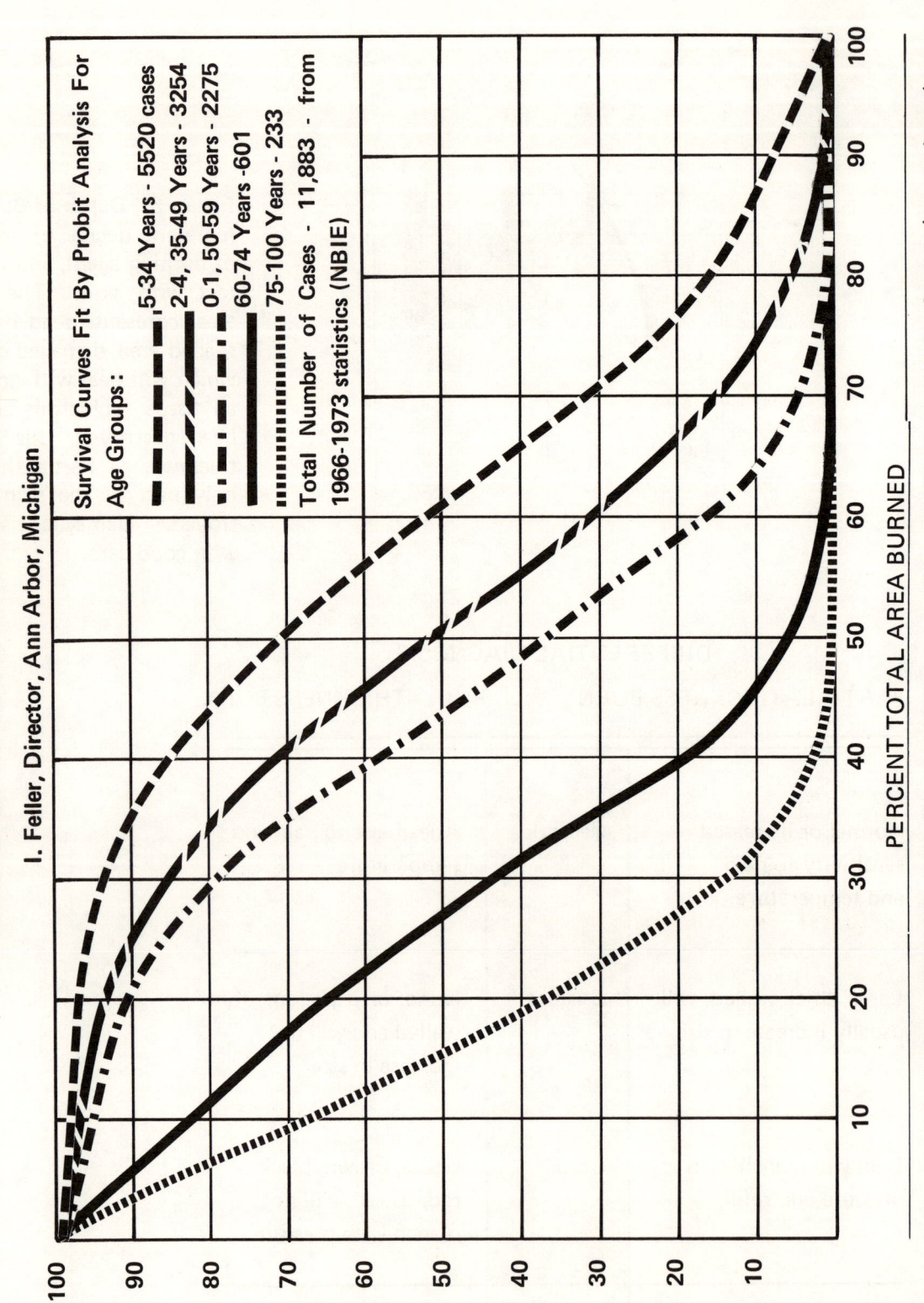

Figure 7. Burn Patient Survival : Age Group vs % Total Area Burned. The two severity factors (age and total area burned) greatly affect chance for survival. It is important, however, to keep in mind that these averages improve with excellence in burn care.

response to infection, leading to septicemia. In the older patient, exacerbation of latent degenerative processes may be fatal.

- Obtain and record the patient's age on the severity sheet.

4. Past Medical History

In patients with a history of chronic or acute disease, such as alcoholism, diabetes, cirrhosis, and heart disease, exacerbation of that disease process by stress of the burn will increase mortality. In a child, the presence of a major anomaly which retards growth, failure to thrive, and congenital heart disease, of course, complicate the burn. Unknown disease may also complicate the burn: e.g., epilepsy or stroke may have caused the accident, and symptoms of these must also be detected.

A dependable history may be given by the adult patient for a few hours after the accident, but after that edema and pain cloud the sensorium. A history is best taken from both the victim and the family.

Obtain a dependable past medical history from the victim and/or the family.

- Obtain and prominently *record* a history of:
  - Recent or past illnesses, chronic and severe.
  - Dependence on life-sustaining medication.
  - Allergies to food or medicine (especially penicillin).
  - Symptoms which may indicate latent and undetected diseases.
  - Events leading to the injury.

5. Part of Body Burned and Concurrent Injury

The part of the body injured is the fifth factor contributing to severity. Burns of the head, neck, and chest lead to increased incidence of pulmonary problems. Burns of the perineum are prone to early infection. Circumferential burns of the neck, chest, and extremity also contribute to severity. A significant injury in addition to the burn also increases severity (for example, electrical injury, skull fracture, serious abdominal injury, or compound fractures). Evidence of such injury must be determined during first aid procedures.

The part of the body injured will affect severity.

- Determine, treat, and record significant concurrent injuries.

6. **Diagnosis of Minor or Major Burn**

The difference between a minor and a major burn is also determined by the above severity factors. For example, a 5% full-thickness burn would be serious for a diabetic patient, but may be only minor for a healthy patient of the same age.

a. **Minor Burn**

It is a minor burn if:

- The full-thickness and partial-thickness loss is less than 10% total body area.
- The patient is more than 4 but less than 35 years of age.
- There is no history of chronic or severe illness.
- There are no significant concurrent injuries (e.g., respiratory damage, fractures, etc.).
- The burn does not include the hands, face, feet, or perineum, and/or no circumferential injury exists.
- It is not an electrical injury.
- Special considerations for a child or dependent (regardless of size of injury):
    - The family can cope with home care.
    - There is no suspicion of abuse or neglect.

b. **Major Burn**

It is a major burn if:

- The wound covers more than 10% total body area.
- The patient is less than 4 years or over 35 years of age.
- There is a medical history positive for chronic or severe illness.
- There are significant concurrent injuries (e.g., respiratory damage, fractures, etc.).
- There are burns of the face, hands, feet, or perineum, and/or circumferential injury.
- It is an electrical injury.
- Special considerations for a child or dependent (regardless of size of injury):
    - The family cannot cope with home care.
    - There is suspicion of abuse or neglect.

c. Level of Care Required

Obviously one very important purpose for determining severity of the burn is to decide where that burn should be treated. A very minor burn can be treated on an outpatient basis either by the family physician or through the hospital Emergency Department. A major burn, however, requires thought further than just a decision to admit. All major burns are not alike, nor are burn care facilities. Major burns are subdivided into moderate, severe, and critical, and the level of care required is based on this. Listed on the EMS Burn Poster (in Box 5) and on page 64 of the text (F. <u>Triage Considerations</u>, 2. <u>Where Should the Patient be Treated?</u>) is a Triage chart, allowing an intelligent, well-founded choice, based on severity, as to what level of burn care that patient requires. Some aspects of major burn treatment are also based on this decision.

The severity of the injury will determine where the patient should be treated.

C. Minor Burn Treatment in the Emergency Department (Box 3, EMS Burn Care Poster)

Wound management is the major consideration for minor burns. There is no need for intravenous fluid therapy or prophylactic antibiotics. Tetanus Toxoid, Tetanus Antitoxin, or Tetanus Immune Globulin (Human), however, is used in all but small partial-thickness burns, based on history of immunization. The basic principles of wound management are cleanliness and comfort. A partial-thickness burn is usually painful because pain fibers in the area of tissue damage are irritated. Analgesics may be necessary before cleaning the involved surface, but care should be taken to avoid oversedation because pain during cleansing helps to prevent excessively rough handling of the tissues. Partial-thickness wounds can be converted to full-thickness loss when added mechanical trauma during cleansing further damages weakened tissues. This can easily occur with infants because their skin is thin.

Partial-thickness injury can be converted to full-thickness loss by over aggressive cleansing and debriding.

After the wound and surrounding areas are gently but thoroughly cleansed of all debris with soap and water and thoroughly rinsed, a dressing is applied. One layer of a saline-moistened roll bandage applied directly to the burned area covered with a moist and then dry Kerlix gauze provides a comfortable occlusive dressing. The patient and family are instructed to change this dressing daily by soaking it off with warm tap water, gently cleansing the wound with soap and

EMERGENT CARE OF THE BURN VICTIM
National Institute for Burn Medicine

water and a thorough rinsing, and then to apply a new one. Dressing changes remove exudate and products of infection, allowing the wound to heal spontaneously. Approximately two weeks are required to heal a partial-thickness wound, and the patient should be followed on an out-patient basis. Appearance of necrotic tissue and/or granulation tissue after the necrotic surface is cleaned indicates a full-thickness wound, usually requiring admission for closure with skin graft.

The patient or family should also be instructed to observe the unburned skin surrounding the wound for evidence of spreading infection during the daily dressing changes. If cellulitis appears, an immediate return visit is indicated for prescription of the proper antibiotic. In most instances, Gram-positive organisms are responsible. Oral antibiotics are usually satisfactory and, of course, more frequent dressing changes with increased soaking periods hasten the control of infection. Oral analgesics are used to minimize the patient's discomfort at any time during the treatment.

Ointments, other topical medications, and expensive dressings are not indicated. There are no chemicals that can restore viability to dead tissue, nor can they speed the body's healing process. Many of the substances used to coat burns have actually increased the injury by their own chemical action on already weakened tissues. *It is not so much what is put on the wound, but how the wound is cared for that is important.*

It is not so much what is put on the wound but skill in providing care that is important.

1. **Wound Care**

   - Cleanse the wound and adjacent areas with cool, sterile saline or tap water and a small amount of surgical detergent.
   - Leave blisters intact if *not* cloudy or leaking.
   - Shave hair from the wound and a 1 inch (or larger) margin around the wound. Clip scalp hair and/or shave the scalp if the wound is on or near the scalp.
   - Debride obviously infected blisters and other loose tissue and debris.
   - Rinse thoroughly with tap water or cool sterile saline.
   - Apply sterile fine mesh gauze to the wound, cover with Kerlix. Moisten both dressings in sterile saline or a topical agent of physician's choice.
   - Cover with a dry outer Kerlix wrap.

Cleanse the wound of all debris (without causing further trauma).

2. **Comfort**

   - Give a systemic analgesic as indicated, e.g., Demerol

(dosage patient-related) for initial care.
- Prescribe a mild analgesic for home care and explain use.

3. **Infection**

    - Determine history of Tetanus coverage.
    - Give Tetanus Toxoid, Tetanus Antitoxin, or Tetanus Immune Globulin (Human) as indicated.
    - Prescribe systemic and topical antibiotics for face, hands, or infected wounds, and give explicit instructions for use.

    Provide Tetanus coverage.

4. **Considerations for Outpatient Care**

    Minor burns are usually treated on an outpatient basis, with the exception of those with suspected or obvious respiratory involvement. If the patient was forced to inhale noxious fumes, gases, or smoke for any length of time, he or she should be admitted for observation regardless of the size of the injury.

    Special consideration must also be given to the ability of the victim or family (if the victim is a child or dependent) to cope with home care. If it is suspected they cannot, the patient must be admitted or Visiting Nurse Association (VNA) follow-up must be constant. Also, if abuse, neglect, or inflicted injury is suspected, the child or dependent must be admitted and the situation evaluated to prevent further occurrence.

    If the patient is treated on an outpatient basis, give *specific* instructions as to the care required to heal the wound and prevent infection. Instruct the patient and/or family to:

    Give clear instructions on the care required to heal the wound.

    - Cleanse the wound (wash with mild soap and tap water) once or twice daily.
    - Rinse the wound thoroughly with cool tap water. (Cleansing may be done in the shower.)
    - Apply dressings as listed in 1. Wound Care.
    - Consult their physician or the ED immediately if there are signs of inflammation (redness, heat, pain, swelling), poor healing, or cellulitis.
    - Continue to take antibiotics for the appropriate time interval.
    - Arrange for return outpatient visits until the wound is healed.

D. Major Burn Care (Box 4, EMS Burn Care Poster)

The life-threatening problems of burn victims are similar to those of any trauma victim. Therefore, immediate first aid attention should be given for breathing, bleeding, and shock.

Once these life-saving measures are taken, fluid therapy to prevent shock and a re-evaluation of respiratory status are in order before burn wound care is considered. Of course, when a team is available, all of these steps in care may progress simultaneously.

A major burn victim requires consideration of all these aspects of care. The decision for extent of wound care required in the Emergency Department is based on the level of specialized burn care required. This decision is made through use of severity factors and use of the Triage chart, on the EMS Burn Poster (in Box 5) and on page 64 of this manual (F. Triage Considerations, 1. Explanation of Triage and 2. Where Should this Patient be Treated?).

1. Respiratory Care

a. Diagnosis

Anticipation of and intervention in respiratory difficulties during emergent period care can reduce the severity of pulmonary complications. Lung involvement may not be apparent immediately post-burn, but should be suspected and treated if the patient has any or all of the following:

- **BURNED IN AN ENCLOSED SPACE AND/OR FORCED TO BREATHE PRODUCTS OF COMBUSTION (E.G., EXPLOSION, HOUSE FIRE).**
- **BLACKENED ORAL AND NASAL MUCOUS MEMBRANES AND/OR SINGED NASAL HAIRS.**
- **BURNS OF THE FACE, NECK, AND/OR CHEST.**
- **OBVIOUS RESPIRATORY DIFFICULTIES.**

If any of these signs are present treatment must be started regardless of the size of the wound.

Any or all of the above indicate impending pulmonary problems. Edema increases insidiously, and within several hours postburn the patient may develop respiratory obstruction.

b. Treatment

If any of the above signs are present, treatment should be started regardless of the extent of burn wound (or even lack of a burn). Upper airway involvement is due to absorption of heat and noxious gases, thus trauma to mucous membrane linings, edema, and possible obstruction. Cold, moist steam (with oxygen) is indicated to humidify incoming air. Insertion of an endotracheal tube is indicated for severe upper airway edema. As edema subsides (within a few days), the obstruction is relieved and the endotracheal tube will be removed.

Lower lung involvement, termed primary pulmonary damage, refers to injury at the alveolar level. Prolonged inhalation of noxious gases and chemicals traumatize deeper lung tissues. Treatment of deep pulmonary involvement is difficult. Tracheostomy is performed if intubation will not resolve airway problems. Blood gas analysis is mandatory. Bronchodilators, steroids, and antibiotics may be indicated to open the airways and to reduce the inflammatory process. Stiff, wet lungs may develop secondary to the injury. A checklist of treatment follows: *not* all are indicated for *every* patient, but each must be considered for every patient with suspected pulmonary problems, even those without burns.

- Provide an open airway.
- Administer precise concentrations of humidified oxygen. Blood gas analysis will be judged in light of FIO_2 (Fractional Inspired Oxygen Concentration).
- Obtain baseline blood gases.
    - Arterial for evaluation of respiratory system.
    - Venous for evaluation of cardio-pulmonary system.
- Measure arterial blood gases $\bar{q}$ 1 to 2 hours.
- Obtain blood for carboxyhemoglobin.
- Obtain a baseline laryngoscopy, if available and if trained to use a fiberoptic laryngoscope.
- Obtain a baseline chest x-ray and then follow-up studies as indicated.
- Administer Aminophyllin if indicated for respiratory distress; wheezing, bronchospasm, etc.
    - Dosage: Aminophyllin:
        - Adults: 250 mg. $\bar{q}$ 6° IV piggyback.
        - Child: dose is weight related.
- Administer steroids in therapeutic doses if indicated for deep lung involvement. Signs of deep lung involvement are:

Administer precise concentrations of humidified oxygen.

EMERGENT CARE OF THE BURN VICTIM National Institute for Burn Medicine

- Carbon deposits on the back of the throat.
- Wheezing.
- Burns of tongue.
- Burned nasal hairs.
- Posterior pharynx swelling.
- Prolonged exposure to smoke in an enclosed space.
- Hacking cough.
- X-ray changes.
- Dosage: SoluCortef 200 mg. IV *Stat* for adult and then 50 mg q̄ 2° until improved, then reduce dose to 25 mg q̄ 2°, within 2 days. (Child dose is weight related.)
- If steroids are begun also:
    - Insert a nasogastric tube (double lumen SUMP) and connect to intermittant suction.
    - Administer antacid 60 ml q̄ 2° per N/G tube for adults, clamp ½ hour, open to suction 1½ hours, repeat.

If resuscitation fluids are necessary, keep the patient with pulmonary problems slighty on the "dry" side.

- If resuscitation fluids are necessary for burn shock, keep the patient with pulmonary problems on the "dry" side of titration. Maintain urine at 20 to 40 ml output per hour for an adult, 10 to 20 ml output per hour for a child.

- **Determine the need for intratracheal intubation as indicated by:**
    - **Progressive stridor.**
    - **Deterioration of arterial gases.**
    - **Extreme anxiety or lethargy (consider hypoxia).**
    - **Difficulty with secretions.**
    - **Questionable respiratory insufficiency when patient must travel long distances to specialized care.**

- Perform tracheostomy *only* when respiratory distress cannot be relieved by intubation.

2. <u>Fluid Therapy</u>

Within a few hours postburn, loss of circulating fluid will cause hypovolemia, which if untreated can lead to hypovolemic shock and death. Advances in the knowledge of fluid therapy now make it possible to successfully resuscitate even the most severely burned victim. However, fluid overload can be an even greater danger and complication of long-term care.

The severe burn results in an outer layer of dead tissue and a deeper band or zone of injured or damaged cells (review Figure 6). The dead tissue is not important to fluid therapy. Fluid does not leave the body, but is leaked out of the bloodstream into the interstitial spaces. Fluid loss through eschar is insignificant compared to the plasma shift. It is in the zone of damaged tissue that fluid shifts, causing hypovolemia (Figure 8). This inflammatory reaction is the body's normal response to trauma. It begins immediately postburn and is profound for the first 24 hours. There is increased capillary permeability in the area of injury, upsetting the delicate balance of extracellular (interstitial and intravascular) fluid. In burns of less than 10 to 20% total body area, depending on other severity factors, the body can compensate for this fluid shift by saving urine, vasoconstriction, etc. However, in larger burns the fluid shift, if untreated, is life-threatening.

FIGURE 8

EDEMA FORMATION

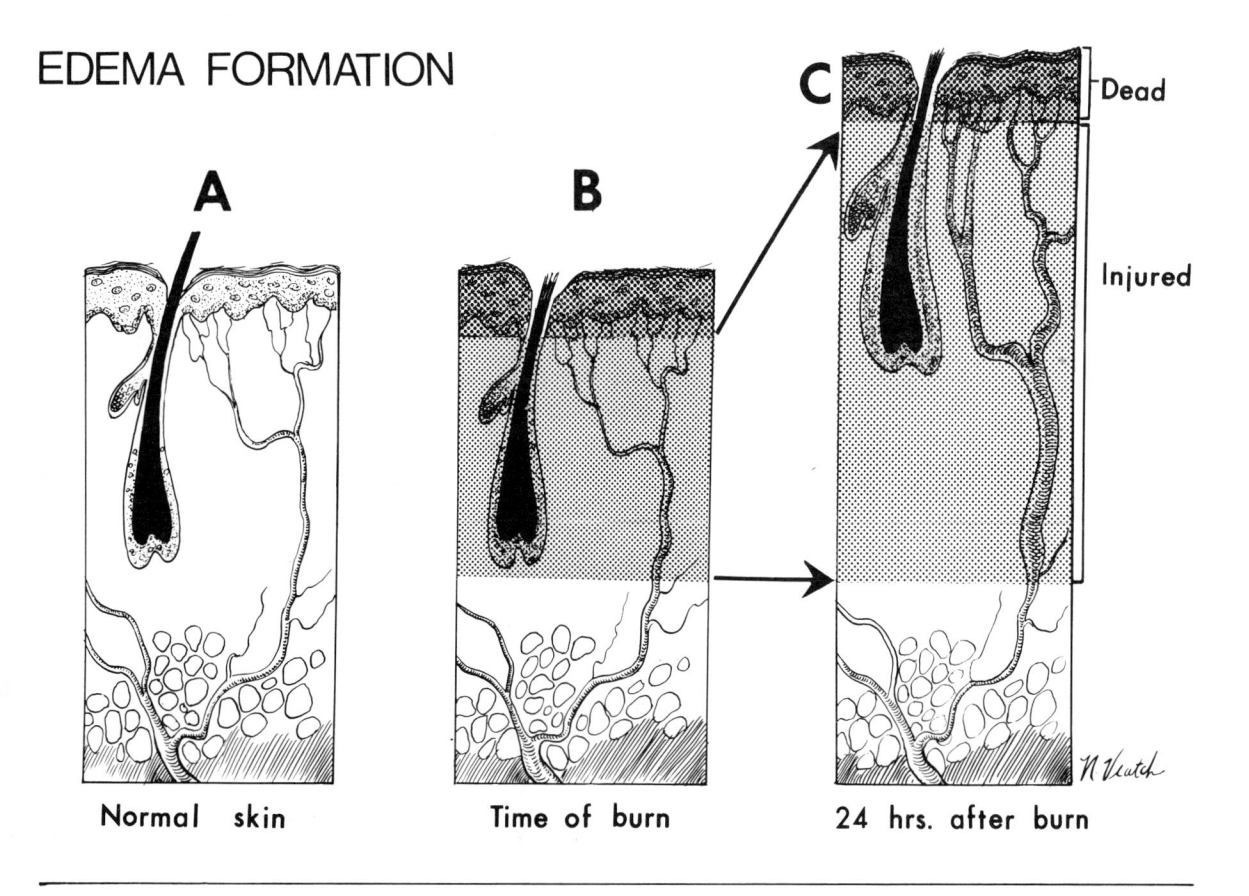

A. Normal skin
B. Time of burn
C. 24 hrs. after burn

Figure 8. Edema Formation. Due to the inflammatory process and increased capillary permeability following deep partial- or full-thickness burns, fluids lost from the vascular spaces enter the injured area. **A.** demonstrates normal skin ; **B.** the depth of the injury at the time of the burn; and **C.** the amount of edema formed in this damaged tissue 24 hours after burn.

EMERGENT CARE OF THE BURN VICTIM

Intravenous fluids similar to those shifted out of the bloodstream, must be given in amounts sufficient to prevent hypovolemic shock, without causing fluid overload and electrolyte imbalance. Ileus is also seen due to the hypovolemic state, and contraindicates oral fluids.

When there is proper fluid replacement, the process gradually reverses. Within a few days the fluid leaked into interstitial spaces returns to the vascular spaces and a profound, spontaneous diuresis occurs, signaling successful resuscitation. (The term resuscitation is used in burn care to denote emergent period treatment which is life-saving, in this instance, successful fluid therapy.) *If excessive fluids have been given, the shift back to vascular spaces may cause hypervolemia, congestive heart failure, and stiff, wet lungs.*

IT IS ESSENTIAL IN FLUID THERAPY RESUSCITATION OF THE BURN VICTIM TO GIVE NOT ONLY THE PROPER TYPE OF FLUID, BUT THE <u>CORRECT</u> AMOUNT.

a. **Which Patients Require Fluid Therapy?**

- All victims of severe burns as diagnosed in this manual require fluid therapy:
    - Any burn over 10% total body area.
    - Any patient under 4 and over 35 years of age.
    - Individual considerations based on severity factors, e.g., infants, aged, dehydrated patients, or those with concurrent injuries.
- Observe patients with smaller burns and give IV fluid only as needed; oral fluids may suffice.
- Keep major burns NPO to reduce the possibility or severity of ileus due to shock.

b. **Method of Fluid Therapy**

A large volume of fluids may be required to resuscitate the major burn; therefore, a large patent veinway is essential.

Insert a large bore transcutaneous IV catheter.

- Insert a large-bore (18 gauge for adults) transcutaneous catheter into a large vein. A central line is not mandatory if not possible; at least do a cutdown of a peripheral vein.

Insert an indwelling urinary catheter.

- Insert an indwelling urinary catheter (Foley) and connect to dependent drainage in any patient with a major burn or burn of the perineum.

c. **What Type of Fluids?**

Fluid lost from the blood stream in **burn shock** is composed of water, electrolytes, and albumin and should be replaced in kind. Red cell loss related to the burn injury is caused by hemolysis and generally approximates only 10% of the total red cell mass. Whole blood is not necessary to resuscitate the victim of a major burn unless there is significant loss of blood from concurrent injuries. Hartmann's solution (lactated Ringer's) is the fluid of choice because the electrolyte balance is similar to that of the blood. Albumin (Human Serum) is added to provide colloid.

Lactated Ringer's is the current solution of choice for resuscitation.

- Give Hartmann's solution (lactated Ringer's) with 25 grams Human Serum Albumin added to each liter.
- Plasma (Fresh Frozen) may also be used if available.

d. **How Much Fluid?**

There are several formulas available to calculate approximate fluid requirements. A formula, however, serves only as a starting point. It is frequently worthwhile for the practitioner new to burn care to evaluate fluid requirements using a formula as a 24 hour yardstick for titration (Figure 9). Rarely is it necessary to give more than a formula indicates. Because the formula cannot possibly consider all of the severity factors, *the patient's individual response is the most important factor in determining fluid requirements.* Keep in mind that resuscitation fluids are also leaked or shifted to interstitial spaces and, therefore, *fluid overload is a constant hazard* of therapy. The parameters most carefully observed are urinary output, blood pressure, pulse, respiratory rate, central venous pressure, weight, and hematocrit.

The patient's individual response is the most important factor in determining fluid requirements.

1) **Parameters of Therapy**

Titration (in burn care, the process of maintaining a predetermined urinary output by IV intake) requires close teamwork. Careful assessment of the patient's response to trauma and treatment is essential. Urinary output, blood pressure, pulse, and respiratory rate, are

FIGURE 9

EXAMPLES OF FORMULAS DEVISED TO STANDARDIZE FLUID THERAPY

EVANS FORMULA:

Dr. Everett Idris Evans introduced the first formula in 1952. He calculated the amount of fluid to be replaced by taking into consideration both the size of the wound and the weight of the patient. Evans recommended that the total estimated amount of colloids and crystalloids (electrolytes) be given during the first 24 hours and one-half of this amount be given during the next 24 hours with appropriate amount of glucose to cover insensible water loss. He was the first to caution that in a burn involving more than 50% the body surface, to avoid overhydration, the fluid requirements should be estimated as though only 50% of the body surface had been burned.

BROOKE FORMULA:

The Brooke Formula was first published in 1953 and is a modification of the Evans Formula. This formula estimates the following requirements for the first 24 hours post-burn:

COLLOIDS: (blood, dextran, plasma) 0.5ml per kg per % of body surface burned.

CRYSTALLOIDS: (lactated Ringer's — Hartmann's solution) 1.5ml per kg of body weight per % of burn.

WATER: (5% Glucose in Water) Dependent on age and size of patient to replace insensible fluid loss.

One-half of the estimated fluid requirements for the first 24 hours is given in the first eight hours, one-quarter of the total in the second eight hours, and one-quarter of the total in the third eight-hour period. The second 24-hour period requirement for colloids and lactated Ringer's — Hartmann's solution is about one-half that for the first 24 hours. In applying this formula to burns of larger than 50%, requirements must be calculated as though only 50% of the body had been burned.

PARKLAND (BAXTER) FORMULA:

The Baxter Formula recommends crystalloid replacement only in the first 24-hour period, given at a replacement rate of 4ml of solution per kilogram of body weight times percentage of burn up to 50% total body area. Half of this amount is given in the first 8 hours. Colloids are not given in the first 24 hours because Baxter etal. did not find a significant reduction in need for crystalloid when colloids were given in the first 24 hours. However, colloids are given in the second 24 hours postburn and are effective in correcting residual plasma volume deficits.

EXAMPLE: 70kg patient, 25 years of age, with 50% total area burned.

FIRST 24 HOURS:

COLLOID SOLUTIONS: (Blood, plasma, plasma expander) None.

ELECTROLYTES: (lactated Ringer's — Hartmann's solution) 4ml x 70kg x 50% = 14,000ml IN FIRST 24 HOURS.

GLUCOSE IN WATER: None (2 liters given in second 24 hour period).

TOTAL 24 HOUR INTAKE: 14,000ml

RATE OF ADMINISTRATION:

1/2	1/4	1/4
First 8 hours	Second 8 hours	Third 8 hours
post burn	post burn	post burn
7,000ml	3,500ml	3,500ml

Figure 9. Formulas for Fluid Therapy. Although fluid therapy should be individualized for each patient, it is useful to complete calculation of a formula as a guideline, and 24 hour double check to prevent copious fluid replacement and overload.

closely monitored. If cardiac involvement is suspected an electrocardiogram is obtained. Initial and daily weights are essential in assessing fluid therapy. The preburn weight is obtained and used as a baseline for daily weight evaluation. Relative hematrocrit values are a clue to the dilution of red blood cells, hence fluid replacement. Red cells do not shift; a concentrated hematocrit is due to burn shock and falls with proper fluid replacement. The hematocrit is obtained in the ED as a baseline and then every 6 hours throughout the emergent period.

- **MONITOR URINARY OUTPUT HOURLY.**
- **MONITOR BLOOD PRESSURE, PULSE, AND RESPIRATIONS EVERY 15 MINUTES.**
- **READ AND RECORD TEMPERATURE EVERY HOUR (IF ELEVATED, READ AND RECORD EVERY 15 MINUTES).**
- **OBTAIN A HEMATOCRIT X 1.**
- **OBTAIN (FROM PATIENT OR FAMILY) AND RECORD THE PATIENT'S PREBURN WEIGHT.**
- **IF POSSIBLE, WEIGH THE PATIENT IN THE EMERGENCY DEPARTMENT.**
- **OBTAIN AN EKG FOR SUSPECTED CARDIAC INVOLVEMENT.**

2) <u>Output</u>

Urinary output is essential in assessing the patient's response to trauma. The amount, content, and color of urine are a guide to fluid replacement. Obviously, the catheter must remain patent for this assessment to be of value. Also keep in mind that urine drains by gravity, and small amounts of urine out are expected immediately postburn. If the urinary drainage tubing is allowed to sag to the floor then back to the collection bottle, a misleading output can be determined and, therefore, an ineffective intake.

The amount of urine measured and recorded each hour is a guide to the amount of fluid to be infused the next hour. An output of 20 to 60 ml of urine per hour for adults and 10 to 30 ml per hour for a pediatric, geriatric, cardiac or respiratory patient indicates *adequate* perfusion of organ systems without systemic overload

The accurate measurment of urinary output each hour is a guide to the amount of IV to infuse the next hour.

of fluids. Maintenance of this volume of urine may require as much as 1,000 ml of fluid in the first one or two hours of care in a previously healthy adult.

Amounts of output over 20 to 60 ml per hour for an adult, or 10 to 30 ml per hour for a child or those with a positive medical history, do NOT indicate "better" resuscitation, but rather invite fluid overload and stiff, wet lungs. If there is no output response to regulating the IV intake within one hour (and the Foley catheter is patent, ascertained by irrigating with a small measured amount of saline), notify the physician.

- Accurately measure and record the amount of urine output hourly.
- Observe output frequently between measurements to assist in regulating IV flow rate and to determine catheter patency.

- **MAINTAIN THE IV INFUSION RATE TO PRODUCE 20 TO 60 ML OF URINE PER HOUR FOR AN ADULT, 10 TO 30 ML PER HOUR FOR A CHILD, GERIATRIC, CARDIAC, OR PATIENT WITH RESPIRATORY INVOLVEMENT.**

- Irrigate the catheter with measured small amounts of normal saline to maintain patency.
- *Note* to those unaccustomed to this method of titration: Maintaining output within these close parameters requires meticulous IV regulation, which is not an immediately simple matter. The amount infused for the previous hour and the present amount of output (along with formula calculation) are your guidelines. Speed or slow the flow rate based on your observations. **Meticulous observation soon relieves anxiety in use of this method.**

3) <u>Physical Examination</u>

When significant past disease or pulmonary damage is suspected, fluid intake is limited to that volume which will provide the lowest acceptable urinary output. The medical history should be reviewed on admission for disease, such as organic heart or primary lung disease which might influence fluid therapy. A thorough knowledge of the patient's medical history is necessary before undertaking extensive fluid therapy.

- Obtain medical history from patient or family.
- Relate physical findings to assessment of therapy.
- A reduced output of 20 ml per hour in the adult, 10 to 20 ml per hour in a child, may be indicated for respiratory involvement or other disease states.

Relate the past medical history and physical findings to assessment of therapy.

4) Hemoglobinuria

Deep tissue injury damages red blood cells (hemolysis), resulting in the release of large amounts of free circulating hemoglobin (hemoglobinemia). When this free hemoglobin passes the basement membrane into the tubules of the kidney, there is the danger of acute tubular necrosis (ATN) and renal failure. Black urine (hemoglobinuria) on catheterization, or in the immediate postburn period, indicates severe hemolysis; an osmotic diuretic is indicated *stat* to flush the tubules. (*Note:* if the patient has not been catheterized on admission, this observation cannot be made. Indwelling urinary catheterization is therefore essential in severe burns.)

Black urine on catheterization indicates severe hemolysis and impending ATN.

- **Give Mannitol intravenously (12.5 gm for adults, less for a child) at first evidence of black urine.**
- **Increase IV intake accordingly.**

3. Medications

a. Infection Control

Routine tetanus coverage is indicated for the burned victim, as for all trauma victims. Wounds should be cultured in the Emergency Department if suspicious. If the circumstances of the injury cause an extremely dirty wound, or if other infectious disease is present, antibiotics may be started in the Emergency Department. Antibiotic coverage will be started or continued in the burn care facility—prophylactic Gram-positive coverage (penicillin or erythromycin) is usually indicated, because Staphylococcus and Streptococcus present on the skin are the first invaders. Other agents specific to bacteria cultures may be given.

- Administer Tetanus Toxoid, Tetanus Antitoxin, or Tetanus Immune Globulin (Human) based on history of immunization.
- Consider need for antibiotic coverage (usually not necessary in the Emergency Department).

b. **Pain Relief**

Any pain relief medication must be given intravenously to be effective during hypovolemic shock.

Although analgesia for pain relief will be necessary, the sensorium should not be dulled. Response to pain is an indicator of other complications, and also serves to prevent too aggressive wound care. Most important, keep in mind that medication given by subdermal or intramuscular route will *not be absorbed* until systemic circulation returns to normal. Because of hypovolemia, the patient will receive no relief from the analgesic, and accumulated, pooled doses may cause cerebral and respiratory depression when circulation is restored. *Pain relief is needed immediately and is given intravenously.* (Tetanus coverage should NOT be given IV. The delay in absorption from a subcutaneous site is acceptable.)

- Give small doses of analgesic of choice (dose weight-related).
    - Adult: 4 to 5 mg Morphine Sulfate IV, q 1°, or Demerol 25 mg IV q̄ 1°.
    - Child: 0.5 mg Dermerol per kg body weight, q̄ 1° IV.
- Observe respirations closely during and after administration of IV narcotics. Do not oversedate!
- Give pain medications INTRAVENOUSLY ONLY both to provide immediate relief and to prevent pooling due to poor circulation.
- **Do not dull the sensorium.**

DO NOT dull the sensorium.

4. Gastrointestinal Considerations.

Shock induces decreased gastric motility and ileus. To prevent distention, nausea, and vomiting, oral fluids are restricted until bowel sounds return. A nasogastric tube is usually inserted in all larger burns, both to deflate the abdomen and to prevent vomiting and possible aspiration.

- Maintain the patient NPO.
- Determine the need for nasogastric drainage.
- Insert a nasogastric tube as indicated and connect to intermittent gastric suction. Do not clamp the nasogastric tube for long periods.
- Irrigate with small measured amounts of saline for patency.
- Provide frequent mouth care and ice chips for comfort.

Maintain the patient NPO.

Provide mouth care for comfort.

5. Laboratory Testing

Baseline blood value determinations are vital to evaluating the patient's state of health on admission and to providing a continuous measurement of response to trauma and therapy. Obtain the following baseline determinations in the Emergency Department:

- WBC and Hematocrit.
- Na, K, CO_2, Cl, BUN, Creatinine.
- Total Protein, A/G ratio, Ca and P.
- PTT, Pro Time or test to indicate bleeder.
- Blood gases (prn).
- Blood type.

Obtain baseline blood tests.

6. Wound Care

The decision as to where the major burn will be treated, and length of time for transfer to that facility should have been made prior to this point in care. Wound care is then based on this decision. <u>Also note that the cause of the burn; thermal, electrical, chemical, etc., does not alter the basic principles of care.</u>

The cause of the burn; thermal, chemical, electrical, etc., does NOT alter the basic principles of wound care.

a. Immediate Transfer to Specialized Care:

If the patient is to be *transferred* to specialized care *within four hours, no burn wound care is necessary.* Wet dressings are not indicated, because they

EMERGENT CARE OF THE BURN VICTIM

National Institute for Burn Medicine

may act as a wick and pull bacteria onto the wound.
- Wrap the patient in a dry, sterile sheet.
- Cover with a blanket for warmth.
- Transport to the burn care facility.

b. **Treatment in Non-Specialized Facility or Delay in Transfer:**

If the patient cannot be transferred within four hours postburn, or will not be given specialized care in a Burn Center, Unit, or Program, *thorough* wound care is essential. The principles of immediate wound care are the same regardless of etiology.

(1) Cleanse the wound, removing all soot, loose tissue, hair, and debris which serve as a source for bacterial growth.

Remove all debris which will provide a source for bacterial growth.

(2) Cleanse areas adjacent to the wound to prevent wicking of bacteria into the burned area (quick bed bath).
(3) Prevent further tissue damage and contamination.
(4) Provide patient comfort.

After systemic therapy is underway, gently but firmly cleanse the wound and adjacent areas of all hair, debris, soot, and loose tissue, *leaving intact blisters undisturbed.* Use the patient's response to pain to prevent overly aggressive cleansing.

If the eyes are involved in the injury, an ophthalmologist should see the patient. It is rare that the cornea or conjunctiva are involved, because the eyelid closes in 1/40th of a second, protecting the eye. Lid burns, however, are frequent when the face is burned.

Use clean technique to cleanse in and around the wound.

- Use clean technique.
- Cleanse the wound and adjacent areas thoroughly with mild surgical soap and tap water or cool, sterile saline.
  - Cleanse the folds of the eyes gently with saline on applicators.
  - Cleanse inside the nares with wet applicators.
  - Cleanse the mouth and oral cavity with mouthwash and swabs.
- If the eyes are involved in the burn:
  - Cover with a moist sterile pad.
  - Call an ophthalmologist as soon as possible.

Obtain an Ophthalmologist consultant for eye injury.

National Institute for Burn Medicine   **EMERGENT CARE OF THE BURN VICTIM**

- Remove all debris, soot, and cut away loose tissue.
- Do not disturb intact blisters.
- Shave *all* hairy areas in and at least a 1 inch margin around the wound.
- Clip scalp hair to 1 inch if in or near the wound.
- *RINSE ALL AREAS THOROUGHLY* with cool tap water or sterile saline.
- Apply sterile saline or topical agent of choice on fine-mesh gauze dressing.
    - Wrapping distal to proximal, apply 1 layer, one wrap circumferentially, overlap, and clip the gauze.
    - Apply the next wrap to slightly overlap, and clip.
    - Continue this wrap method until all wound areas are covered. (Figure 10.)
    - Do not wrap unburned areas.
- Hold fine mesh gauze in place with Kerlix also moistened in the topical agent of physician's choice. Wrap in same manner as fine mesh gauze.
- Apply a continuous dry Kerlix as the outer dressing—also wrapped distal to proximal.
- *Cover the patient with a sterile bath blanket for warmth (to prevent chilling).*
- Transfer to a clean, dry stretcher, or change linen after wound care.

Shave all hair from the wound.

Rinse the wound throughly.

No two burn surfaces should touch. Apply fine mesh gauze between fingers, toes, buttocks, etc.

Figure 10. Dressing Application. A. Wrap moist fine mesh gauze, (distal to proximal) one layer overlap and clip. Second wrap slightly overlapping first; **B.** apply moist kerlix as second layer in same manner; and **C.** apply continuous dry kerlix to hold moist layers in place (third layer).

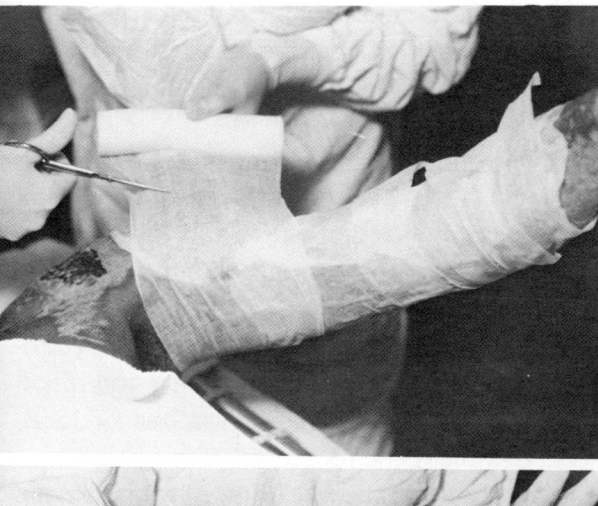

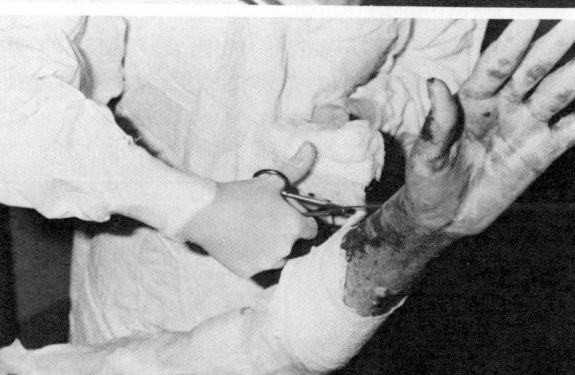

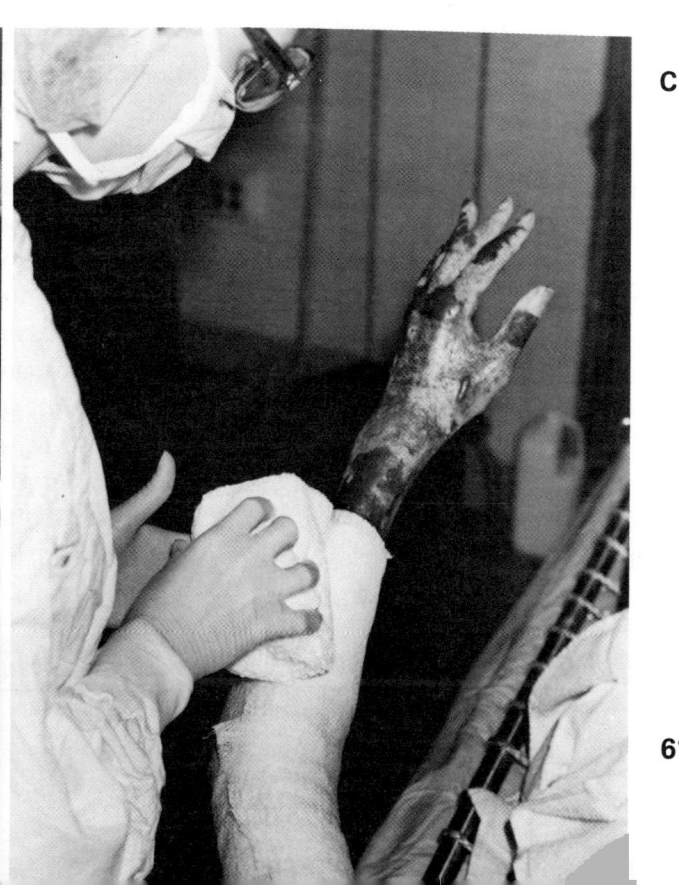

7. **Summary Charting**

   A special summary chart has been developed (Figure 11) to aid in coordinating therapy. This chart permits the accurate hourly recording of the many observations which prove useful in evaluating the patient's course, and serves as a guide to therapy throughout the emergent period of care. If at all possible this or a similar chart should be adopted for Emergency Department use for burn patients. A copy of this chart should accompany the patient to specialized care.

8. **Mass Casualties**

   The primary consideration in dealing with multiple burn admissions is to assess all patients in light of the severity factors, provide first aid, and begin fluid therapy. Wound care can be accomplished after life-saving measures have been taken.

E. **Emergency Department Care of Frostbite**

   Care of the frostbite victim in the Emergency Department requires special attention. As always the first consideration is evaluation of the patient's general condition. Of prime concern is the degree of hypothermia present. Body heat loss and general cooling, with exhaustion of core temperature, may lead to death. Body temperature below 94° (F) results in loss of homothermic control. Unrelieved heat loss can result in coma and cardiopulmonary failure even before body temperatures reach 88° (F).

   The resuscitation technique recommended by W.J. Mills, Jr.[†] is **rapid thawing** of the patient with warm packs and blankets, or by immersion in a hydrotherapy tub at a temperature of 100 to 103° (F). Whenever the rapid thawing method is used, it is essential to include general systemic care: Oxygen, IV fluids, intubation, tracheostomy, defibrillation, baseline electrolyte studies, etc. as *indicated*. Pre-existing trauma and blood loss, disease, alcoholism, and/or anoxia, generalized or local, may well complicate treatment and recovery.

   Rapid thawing in a warm bath will bring a rapid dramatic response in the patient. *Metabolic changes may also be rapid and dramatic.* Thawed tissues release end products of meta-

Rapid thawing treatment will bring a rapid dramatic metabolic response. Systemic monitoring is essential.

[†]W.J. Mills, Jr., Frostbite and Hypothermia, a Discussion of the Problem and a Review of an Alaskan Experience, Alaska Medicine (15:2), March 1973, pp. 26-59.

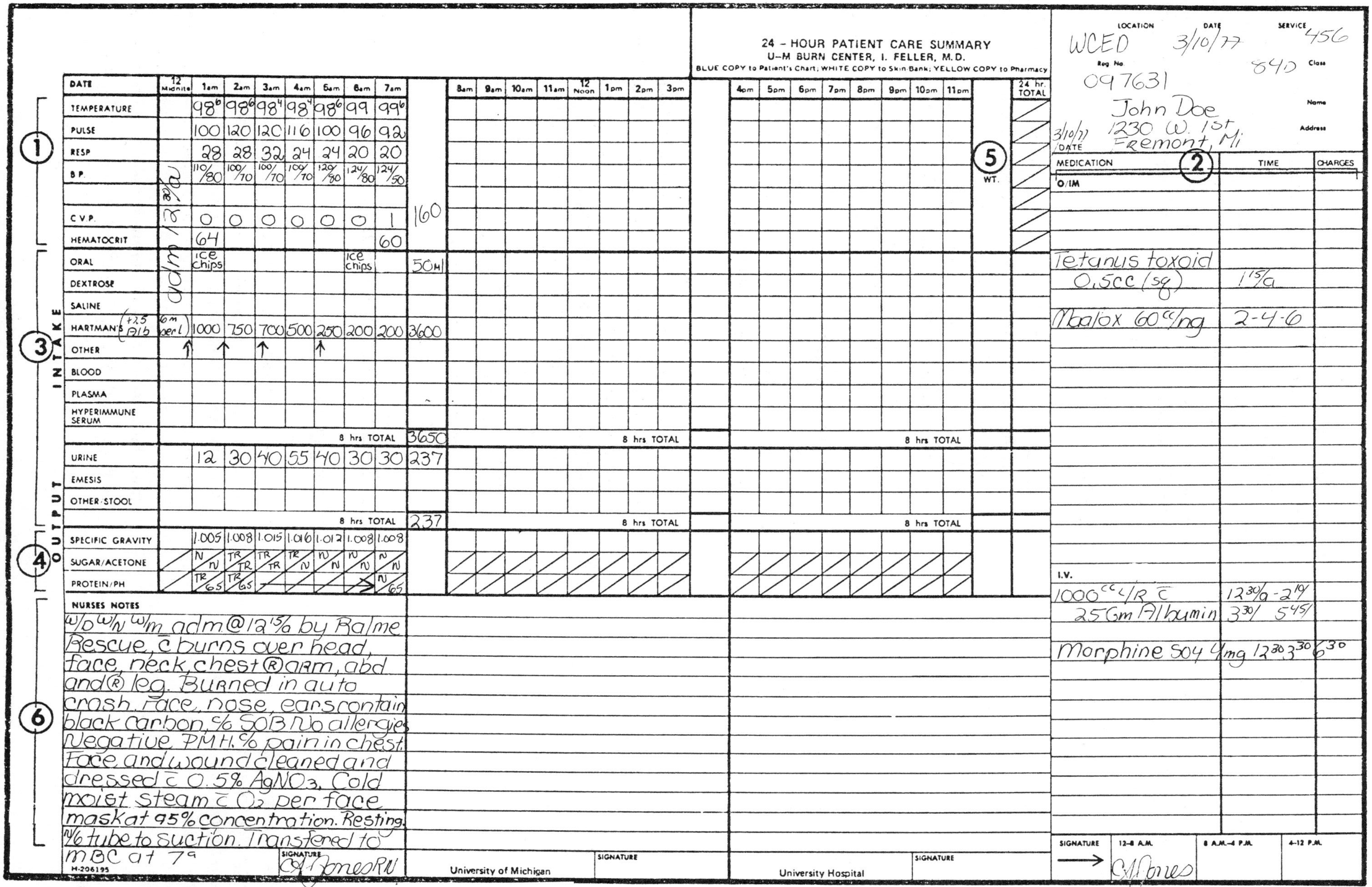

National Institute for Burn Medicine   **EMERGENT CARE OF THE BURN VICTIM**

Figure 11. 24-hour Patient Care Summary. Use of this chart allows not only accurate recording of data essential to assessing the patient's condition, but also serves as a guide to parameters to be considered in providing excellence in care; **1.** Vital Signs and Hematocrit, **2.** Medications, **3.** and **4.** Intake and Output, **5.** Weight, and **6.** Nurses notes.

EMERGENT CARE OF THE BURN VICTIM

bolism, and sudden metabolic acidosis can result in death from ventricular fibrillation (within 1 to 3 hours after thawing). The same result is only delayed (48 to 72 hours) if slow thawing at room temperature is employed. Initial care then is directed to rapid thawing and to prevention of complications resulting from thawing. Monitoring of electrolytes (especially potassium), pH, cardiac status, blood gases, etc. must begin immediately and treatment modified as indicated.

Monitor electrolytes, pH, cardiac status and blood gases closely during rapid thawing.

Rapid Thawing Treatment:

- Protect the frozen part from trauma. Do not remove loose tissue. Do not rub, chafe, or massage frozen part. Do not use ice or cold water applications.
- Thaw the frozen part, or warm the cooled body *rapidly* using constant temperatures of 100 to 103° (F), either in a whirlpool bath or using warm wet packs. **Temperature should *never* exceed 112° (F) or 44.5° (C).**
- Thawing is complete when there is flushing of the DISTAL tip of the thawed part.
- Give a pain medication or sedative (not so as to dull sensorium) because thawing is painful.
- *Do not* use rapid rewarming if part has been thawed previously.
- Monitor and record blood pressure, pulse, respiration, and temperature frequently (q 15 min. to 1 hour).
- Obtain EKG monitoring as indicated (if available use continuous monitor).
- Wrap wounds in dry sterile dressings.
    - *Do not* break blisters or debride loose tissue.
    - Protect injured area from further trauma.
- Wrap the patient in a clean, dry sheet.
- Cover with a blanket for warmth.
- Transfer to a specialized burn care facility.

F. **Triage Considerations (Box 5, EMS Poster)**

1. **Explanation of Triage**

Excellence in care begun in the Emergency Department should continue in the proper specialized burn care facility.

As important as Emergency Department care is to the severely burned individual, equally valuable is ensuring that this excellence in care will continue. If at all possible, the patient should be transferred (triaged) to a specialized burn care facility *promptly*. A frequent misconception is that the severely burned victim is too ill to be transferred. With proper first aid, the patient remains in relatively good condition at least 24 hours postburn. Once the patient has received care in the Emergency Department, as described in this text, arrangements should be made to transfer that victim to specialized burn care.

Just as all burns are not alike, burn care facilities also vary in their ability and resources necessary to provide proper care. To describe precisely the spectrum of burn treatment, three levels of specialized burn care have been defined in order of increasing specialization: (1) Burn Program, (2) Burn Unit, and (3) Burn Center. They are defined as follows:

- *Burn Programs* are found in the hospital which has no specialized facilities or areas for burn care, but in which a consistent plan, conducted by an interested and experienced physician (or jointly by many physicians) is followed for management of burns (e.g., Burn Service). As a measure of experience, it is assumed that the physician is treating at least 25 burns per year.
- A *Burn Unit* is a burn program conducted in a specialized facility which is used only for burns, manned by trained burn personnel. It is assumed that this facility has at least 6 beds and at least 50 patients are admitted and treated each year.
- A *Burn Center* is a specialized facility providing comprehensive burn patient care with additional emphasis on teaching and research. It is assumed that this facility has at least 10 beds and treats at least 100 acute patients annually. A team of highly trained burn specialists staff the Burn Center.

Just as all burn victims are not alike, burn care facilities also vary in their ability to provide care. As shown in Figure 12, moderate burns should be treated in a burn program, severe burns in a burn unit, and critical burns only in a burn center.

2. <u>Where Should the Patient be Treated? (Decision to Triage)</u>

Based on the severity factors, a decision should be made as to which level of burn care the patient requires. The chart in Figure 12 directs this choice of specialized burn care based on severity of the victim's injury. (Also see Box 5, EMS Poster.) The patient's family should also be consulted and aware of triage and transfer arrangements. The extent of wound care provided in the Emergency Department is also based on this decision.

The level of care required is based on the severity of the injury.

3. <u>Information to Give the Burn Care Facility Regarding the Transfer</u>

A smooth transition of care from the Emergency

EMERGENT CARE OF THE BURN VICTIM — National Institute for Burn Medicine

FIGURE 12

RECOMMENDATIONS FOR BURN CARE FACILITY TRIAGE

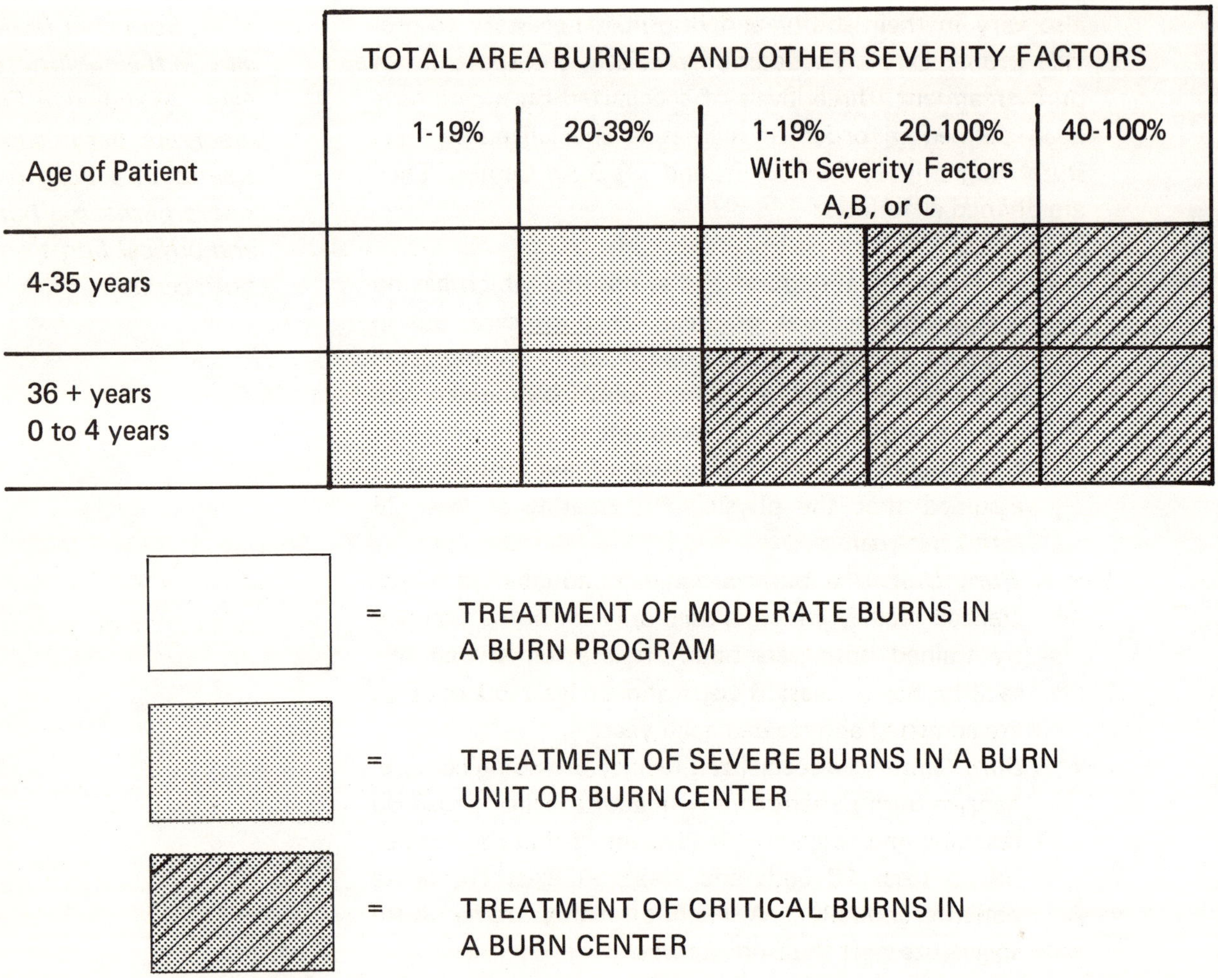

Age of Patient	TOTAL AREA BURNED AND OTHER SEVERITY FACTORS				
	1-19%	20-39%	1-19% With Severity Factors A,B, or C	20-100% With Severity Factors A,B, or C	40-100%
4-35 years	(moderate)	(severe)	(severe)	(critical)	(critical)
36 + years / 0 to 4 years	(severe)	(severe)	(critical)	(critical)	(critical)

☐ = TREATMENT OF MODERATE BURNS IN A BURN PROGRAM

▦ (dotted) = TREATMENT OF SEVERE BURNS IN A BURN UNIT OR BURN CENTER

▨ (hatched) = TREATMENT OF CRITICAL BURNS IN A BURN CENTER

A. **Part of Body Burned:** A burn of the face, neck, and/or chest, burns of hands, feet, perineal area, or a circumferential wound.

B. **Past Medical History:** A medical history affecting present health (e.g., diabetes, heart disease, etc.).

C. **Concurrent Injury:** An injury in addition to the burn (e.g., electrical injury, pulmonary damage, skull fracture, severe abdominal injury, etc.).

Figure 12 demonstrates the criteria for determining the level of specialized burn care required by the burned patient based on the severity of injury.

Prepared by the National Institute for Burn Medicine
909 East Ann Street, Ann Arbor, Michigan 48104

Department to the specialized burn care facility is also essential. It is sad indeed when excellent care has been initiated at the scene of the accident and continued in the Emergency Department, only to be erased through careless handling in transfer. The burn care facility should be properly notified, giving the following data:

- **NAME OF PATIENT.**
- **AGE.**
- **SEX.**
- **CAUSE AND TIME OF BURN.**
- **ESTIMATED PERCENTAGE OF BODY BURNED AND INVOLVED AREAS.**
- **CONCURRENT INJURIES.**
- **MEDICAL HISTORY.**
- **TREATMENT INSTITUTED IN THE EMERGENCY DEPARTMENT.**
- **PRESENT CONDITION OF PATIENT.**
- **METHOD OF TRANSPORT AND EXPECTED TIME OF ARRIVAL.**

Send with the patient a record of therapy, patient's responses, and referring physician's name and phone number. Inform the family or friends of the victim as to transfer plans and assist them to make their plan for accompanying the patient.

Send along a record of treatment, patient's responses, and name and phone number of referring physician and hospital.

4. **Therapy Enroute to a Burn Care Facility**

All care initiated in the Emergency Department must be continued during transportation to the specialized burn care facility. A copy of the ED chart listing all treatments and medications should also accompany the patient. The following checklist should be used to ensure continuity of care through transport.

a. **Respiratory Support**

- Maintain a patent airway.
- If the patient is entubated, *ensure proper placement* and a patent endotracheal tube.
- Suction upper airway as needed.
- Continue humidified oxygen and/or other respiratory assistance.

Maintain a patent airway and adequate oxygen intake.

b. **Fluid Therapy**

- **Maintain a patent IV line.**

Maintain a patent IV and proper intake.

EMERGENT CARE OF THE BURN VICTIM National Institute for Burn Medicine

- Continue IV infusion of lactated Ringer's to produce:
  - 20 to 60 ml of urine per hour for adults.
  - 10 to 30 ml per hour for children, geriatrics, and those with cardiac or respiratory problems.
- Give no oral fluids.

c. **Urinary Output**

Maintain a patent urinary catheter and proper amount of output.

- Measure hourly urines (observe output for amount and color, frequently).
- Maintain a patent urinary catheter.
- Report black urine immediately.

If the patient will arrive at a specialized care facility within the hour, treatment for hemoglobinuria may be delayed. If radio contact is maintained and arrival is delayed, Mannitol may be given on physician's orders for hemoglobinuria (see page 57).

d. **Gastrointestinal Support**

- Prevent aspiration (head of bed elevated if blood pressure 100/- or over).
- Maintain the patient NPO.

Maintain the patient NPO.

- Continue nasogastric suction, with intermittent, low pressure enroute. Do not clamp the NG tube, because this will defeat its purpose. If necessary (no suction available), wrap the end of the NG tube in a "baggie".
- Provide mouth care and/or ice chips sparingly.

e. **Wound Care**

Keep the patient warm.

- Keep patient *warm;* cover with a blanket.

f. **Pain Relief**

- Give a pain medication IV before transportation. (Chart medicine, dosage, and route.)
- Do not oversedate.
- Gently restrain the difficult patient.

Assess the patients condition frequently.

g. **Assess Condition of Patient**

- Check blood pressure, pulse, and respiration q̄ 15

minutes, more or less frequently as indicated.
- Elevate the <u>foot</u> of the bed if blood pressure is below 100/-.

h. **Emotional Support**

- Every comfort and safety consideration must be given the patient.
- Talk *to* the patient not *about* him/her.
- Make him/her comfortable and encourage rest.
- Provide reassurance as needed.

Talk with the patient not about him.

5. **Transition to a Specialized Burn Care Facility**

Upon arrival at the specialized burn care facility continuity of care should take place until relieved by trained burn care staff.

- Continue therapy until instructed to stop.
- Give the following information to the physician or nurse receiving the patient :
  - Name and address of victim.
  - Cause and description of accident.
  - Condition of the patient during transport.
  - Care given during transport.
- Give a copy of the medical record from the referring ED, and place and name of referring physician.

Continue therapy until relieved by the burn team.

ATTENTION TO DETAIL MAY NOT ONLY MEAN THE DIFFERENCE BETWEEN LIFE AND DEATH BUT ALSO REDUCE THE SEVERITY OF COMPLICATIONS.